HEART HEALTH FOR WOMEN

Felicity Smart, the author of this book, has edited many popular health publications. She is now a medical writer and this is her third book. Her previous two, *The Woman's Guide to Surgery* (with Tim Coltart) and *Fibroids* (with Professor Stuart Campbell), are also published by Thorsons.

Dr Diana Holdright, the medical adviser to this book, is a Senior Registrar in Cardiology practising at University College Hospital and the Middlesex Hospital, London. Previously she worked at the London Chest Hospital, the Royal Brompton National Heart & Lung Hospital and the National Heart & Lung Institute, where she carried out research into heart disease in women. She also lectures on the subject and writes for medical textbooks and journals.

HEART HEALTH
FOR WOMEN

Felicity Smart
Medical Adviser: Dr Diana Holdright

Thorsons
An Imprint of HarperCollins*Publishers*

Thorsons
An Imprint of HarperCollins*Publishers*
77–85 Fulham Palace Road,
Hammersmith, London W6 8JB
1160 Battery Street,
San Francisco, California 94111–1213

Published by Thorsons 1995
1 3 5 7 9 10 8 6 4 2

Illustrations produced by the Department of Photography,
Printing and Design at UMDS Guy's and St Thomas's Medical
and Dental School.
Artist: Susanna Nasskau

A catalogue record for this book is available
from the British Library

ISBN 0 7225 2992 9

Printed in Great Britain by
HarperCollinsManufacturing Glasgow

CONTENTS

Acknowledgements vii

Foreword ix

Introduction xi

1 How Your Heart Works 1

2 What Can Go Wrong with Your Heart 16

3 Why Does Heart Disease Develop? 27

4 Investigating Heart Problems 44

5 Treatments 63

6 Recovery and Rehabilitation 101

7 Having a Healthy Heart 116

References and Further Reading 157

Useful Addresses 164

Index 169

Acknowledgements

We thank the following for their contributions to the writing of this book:

Professor Stuart Campbell, Head of Obstetrics & Gynaecology, King's College Hospital, London.
Dr Ian McLean Baird, Medical Spokesman, British Heart Foundation.
Dr Henry Purcell, Senior Research Fellow in Cardiology, Royal Brompton National Heart & Lung Hospital, London.
Dr Anne Charlton, Director, Cancer Research Campaign, University of Manchester.
Dr Mark Bushnell, General Practitioner.
Andy Cox, Senior Nurse Manager, Transplant Clinic, Harefield Hospital.
Carole Flowers, Clinical Nurse Specialist, Cardiac Rehabilitation, London Chest Hospital.
Miranda Buckley, Social Worker, Royal Brompton National Heart & Lung Hospital, London.
Lorna Rappaport, Gay Sutherland and Mary Hayward, Health Behaviour Unit, Institute of Psychiatry, London.
Michele Turney, Production Editor, Thorsons.

Felicity Smart personally thanks Laura Burbidge, Joy Langridge, Liz Versleys, Susanna Nasskau, Dr Gill Shepherd, Nicola Furber, Gisela Taylor and especially Tim Smart, husband and life-support.

FOREWORD

Coronary heart disease has only recently become recognized as a major cause of disability and death among women. Previously, it was considered to be mainly a male problem because it affects large numbers of men from a younger age. In women, however, the incidence rises from the time of the menopause, but risk factors earlier in their lives influence its development, so women of all ages need to be well-informed of the dangers.

Fortunately, this much-neglected area of female health is rapidly becoming the focus of medical research, yet there is still a lack of information specifically for women on the causes, symptoms, treatments and – most importantly – the prevention of heart disease. This book explains in straightforward terms how women can reduce their risk. It describes the treatments available should any problems arise, and advises on rehabilitation.

Heart disease is one of the most frightening disorders, but much can be done both to prevent and alleviate it. This book will help communication between a woman and her doctor. It will also encourage women to have a healthier heart for life – and is therefore essential reading for every woman who cares about her heart.

Professor Sir Magdi Yacoub

INTRODUCTION

'A silent epidemic' is how coronary heart disease in women has been described. It is the largest single killer of women, claiming more lives than lung cancer and all the female cancers put together. Yet women's health is still seen very much in terms of their reproductive system because so much more is known about how it functions. There is thus little information for women on how to protect themselves from heart disease, and on the treatments available should they develop it.

Why has the importance and severity of heart disease in women gone unrecognized for so long? As Professor Sir Magdi Yacoub has pointed out in the Foreword to this book, heart disease and heart attacks start to strike large numbers of men at a younger age; this is the major reason why heart disease has been seen as mainly a male problem.

Women are thought to be protected by the hormone oestrogen, which supports fertility before the menopause. This protection, however, is not absolute. It is estimated that of all deaths from heart attacks in women under 65, about a quarter occur in those under 45, and there are fears that the number will grow. After the menopause, when oestrogen levels fall, women become as vulnerable to heart disease as men. Coronary heart disease affects about one in nine women aged between 45 and 64 and about one in three over the age of 65, equalling the incidence in men.

Ultimately, it kills more women than men.

It is not just the threat to life that is significant, as people with heart disease can suffer pain, fear and a diminished quality of life. And the disease process – the furring-up of arteries – is the same as leads to strokes, the other major cause of death and disability.

The later onset of heart disease in the majority of women, and the lack of information about it, has meant that women – and their doctors – are less aware of the threat and therefore less likely to consider it a risk. Women, however, are more likely than men to have warning symptoms before a heart attack occurs. This should have given us an advantage, enabling those affected to be treated earlier, but until very recently this has not been the case.

To complicate matters, symptoms in women are not always as typical of heart disease as they are in men, and so may be misinterpreted, particularly in a younger woman. Women are also more likely than men to suffer from chest pain that is not due to heart disease. Furthermore, the standard diagnostic tests used are less accurate in women. As if this weren't enough, until recently women have also been thought to gain less benefit than men from invasive treatments, such as angioplasty and coronary artery bypass grafting.

There is now growing recognition of the risk to women and acceptance that if they are treated earlier in the disease process, the long-term benefits can be as great for them as for men. This means that more thorough investigation of symptoms is being considered worthwhile, and so the outlook for women with heart disease is improving.

But prevention is as vital as being treated. In this book, we not only fully explain the causes, symptoms, investigation and treatment of heart disease, we also offer comprehensive advice which will help both in prevention and recovery. It is also a book that will help those who are caring for a woman with heart disease.

The fear that many more younger women will become vulnerable is due to the increasing numbers who are smoking. This major risk factor can override any female advantage earlier in life and, as everyone must know, is also implicated in causing cancer. An unhealthy lifestyle at any age increases the likelihood of developing heart disease.

Virtually all of us are probably aware of how important it is not to smoke, and to eat healthily, take regular exercise and reduce stress. There is no lack of publicity giving us this sound advice which, if followed, will improve every aspect of our health. Even so, the message often goes unheeded. We examine the reasons why this is the case and make some constructive suggestions, since self-help is vital to prevention and recovery.

A very encouraging area of medical research may offer women further help. This concerns hormone replacement therapy (HRT). By replacing oestrogen after the menopause, when women become most at risk of heart and artery disease, HRT may continue the protection this hormone is thought to provide in younger women. HRT is currently given to help relieve menopausal symptoms and to protect the bones from the effects of ageing. But its most important role may prove to be in protecting women from heart disease and strokes. We explain the latest findings so that women who are considering HRT can discuss this aspect with their doctor.

The heart is complex, with great physical and emotional significance. This is the first book devoted entirely to the female heart. In writing it, I realized how much the information is needed by all women and I have endeavoured to present it in a clear and helpful way. This book would not have been possible, however, without the specialist medical knowledge and expertise of my collaborator, Cardiologist Dr Diana Holdright, whose generous help I greatly appreciate. The interest shown by Professor Sir Magdi Yacoub has given us both tremendous encouragement. I am grateful to John Gold for his advice on complementary therapies. Jane Graham-Maw, Publishing Director at Thorsons, had the foresight to commission the book and the patience to support us through a demanding but immensely worthwhile undertaking.

We sincerely hope that this book will help you to understand how, and why, heart disease affects women, and enable you to take the necessary steps to keep your heart in good health, or to restore it to the best possible health.

Felicity Smart

Chapter 1
HOW YOUR HEART WORKS

To care for your heart, first you need to understand it. Knowing how your heart works will help you to maintain its health and, should any problems arise, will enable you and your doctor to discuss them more easily. For women needing treatment, an understanding of the heart can encourage healing and recovery.

So how does this most vital of vital organs keep you alive? What makes it beat? Why does it beat faster at some times than others? And – since this is a book for women – is your heart any different to a man's?

The Female Heart

It would be reasonable to think that a woman's heart must somehow be unlike a man's, simply because women differ physically (and some would say mentally and emotionally) from men in a number of ways. Yet the female heart is the same as the male, albeit smaller, reflecting the usual difference in body size. But the study of 'gender differences' in relation to heart disease is a much-neglected area which is now becoming increasingly recognized as important. The following chapters reveal the latest findings on how women may differ from men in their susceptibility to heart disease and in their response to treatment.

1

The Structure of the Heart

The heart is designed to be the powerhouse of your body, continually driving the circulation of the blood to all the cells which make up the tissues, muscles and organs. Oxygen and nutrients essential for their function and repair are carried in the bloodstream, as are hormones (the body's 'chemical messengers', *see page 11*). Carbon dioxide and other waste products are removed from the cells by the blood. Just keeping warm also depends on an efficient circulation, like a good central-heating system. You are alive because your heart makes these vital activities possible.

The heart is located in your chest between the lungs, as you are no doubt aware. One third is positioned underneath the sternum (the central breastbone) and two thirds slanting to your left. The apex (its lowest point) is beneath the left breast. The illustrations show its shape, which is only a little like the romantic image of a heart.

From childhood, the heart increases in size as part of normal development until about the late teens or early 20s, when it stops growing. It may become slightly larger if regular strengthening exercise is taken (*see Chapter 7*), but any significant enlargement of the heart in an adult indicates problems. The average adult heart measures about 12 cm (4¾ in) lengthways and 8–9 cm (3–3½ in) across at its broadest part, while its depth from front to back is around 6 cm (2½ in). In men it weighs around 280–340 g (10–12 oz); in women it is less, about 230–280 g (8–10 oz).

Most of the heart is made of a unique muscle called the myocardium which is responsible for the pumping action we experience as the heartbeat. The heart is, in fact, a dual pump because the circulatory system has two major parts: the 'systemic' circulation which supplies the whole body except the lungs, and the 'pulmonary' circulation to (and from) the lungs. In order to accommodate both, the heart is hollow inside and divided in half down the middle by a muscular wall called the septum. Each half is further divided into an upper chamber called an atrium and a larger, lower one called a ventricle. Inside the heart there are thus four distinct hollow chambers. The left and right atria receive the blood, and the corresponding ventricles below them act as pumps, propelling the blood upwards into vessels leading from the top of the heart to the body or lungs. The circulatory system is also known as the cardiovascular system, which comes from *kardia*, the Greek for heart, and *vascularis*, Latin for vessels.

Your Heart and Lungs

Your cardiovascular and respiratory systems are intimately connected, which means that your heart and lungs depend on each other. The purpose of the respiratory system is to provide the constant supply of oxygen needed by the body cells for them to function, and to remove waste carbon dioxide from them. Respiration is better known simply as breathing.

You breathe in air containing vital oxygen, and this passes into millions of tiny air sacs in your lungs called alveoli. The oxygen then diffuses into blood vessels surrounding the alveoli which connect with the pulmonary veins, the vessels which carry the oxygen-rich blood to the left side of your heart, where the systemic circulation to your body begins.

The Circulation to the Body

The left atrium receives the oxygenated blood (which is bright red), then contracts to expel it into the left ventricle below. From there it is pumped upwards into the main blood vessel leading from the heart, the artery called the aorta, which carries it to all parts of the body through its various branches.

These branches lead into smaller vessels (arterioles), which connect with a network of tiny vessels, called capillaries. Oxygen and nutrients pass through the very thin walls of the capillaries, taking carbon dioxide and other waste products from the cells in exchange. The deoxygenated blood (now dark red without oxygen) is transferred onwards via the capillaries to small vessels (venules) connected to veins (larger vessels responsible for returning blood to the heart). These lead into the superior and inferior venae cavae, the two main veins which carry blood to the right side of the heart, where the pulmonary circulation to the lungs starts.

The Circulation to the Lungs

The blood enters the right atrium and is then transferred to the right ventricle below, from where it is pumped upwards into the pulmonary artery leading to the lungs. On arrival, another exchange takes place through the blood vessels surrounding the alveoli: waste carbon dioxide is given up and breathed out. More oxygen then diffuses into the blood vessels and, again, oxygenated blood is returned by the pulmonary veins to the left side of the heart, where it re-enters the systemic circulation to the body (*see illustrations*).

To function efficiently, both sides of the heart must contract and relax together and pump the same volume of blood. More force is required, however, to circulate blood to the body than to the lungs, which is why the left side of the heart is more muscular than the right.

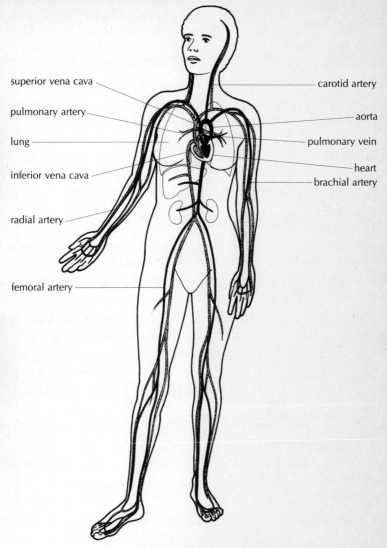

superior vena cava

pulmonary artery

lung

inferior vena cava

radial artery

femoral artery

carotid artery

aorta

pulmonary vein

heart

brachial artery

The circulatory system carries oxygenated blood (shown in black) from the left side of the heart via the arteries to supply all the body's tissues and organs with oxygen and nutrients. Deoxygenated blood (shown in grey) is returned via the veins to the right side of the heart, where it is circulated to the lungs to be reoxygenated and then returned to the left side of the heart.

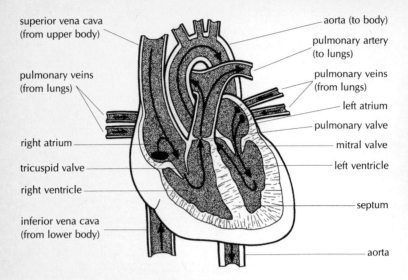

superior vena cava
(from upper body)

aorta (to body)

pulmonary artery
(to lungs)

pulmonary veins
(from lungs)

pulmonary veins
(from lungs)

left atrium

pulmonary valve

right atrium

mitral valve

tricuspid valve

left ventricle

right ventricle

septum

inferior vena cava
(from lower body)

aorta

Inside the heart, blood enters both atria. The left receives oxygenated blood from the lungs via the pulmonary veins; the right receives deoxygenated blood from the body via the two venae cavae. It is pumped through the valves (the mitral and the tricuspid) into the ventricles below, and then pumped upwards. From the left it passes through the aortic valve (not shown) into the aorta, leading to the body. From the right, it enters the pulmonary artery through the pulmonary valve which leads to the lungs.

A One-way System

Because the cardiovascular system is one-way, blood must be prevented from flowing backwards. Within the heart there are four valves that stop this happening: two between the atria and ventricles; and two controlling the exits from the ventricles, one leading to the aorta on the left and the other to the pulmonary artery on the right.

These valves have flaps which open and close in response to the pumping action of the heart. The valve between the left atrium and ventricle has two flaps (or cusps) like a bishop's mitre, and so is known as the mitral valve. Between the right atrium and ventricle there is a valve with three flaps (cusps), the tricuspid valve. Both the aortic and pulmonary valves also have three cusps. These cusps open in one direction only to allow blood through and then snap firmly shut. For your heart to function effectively as a pump, these valves must be in good working order.

When blood has been pumped out of your heart into the circulation, it must be kept flowing in one direction only. It is therefore propelled into the aorta, the main artery to the body, at a high enough pressure to keep it moving. The aorta and its branches have thick, elastic, muscular walls to withstand this pressure. They continue to push the blood forwards between heartbeats and also even out the pressure, so that it is relatively constant by the time blood reaches the arterioles. By the time oxygenated blood has circulated and is being returned to the heart in a deoxygenated state by the veins (except by the pulmonary veins, which carry oxygenated blood from the lungs to the heart), pressure has fallen and it is travelling much more slowly. The walls of the veins are thinner and less muscular than those of arteries; the blood is kept flowing forwards by one-way valves in the veins and by pressure on the walls from the movement of muscles in your arms and legs. To maintain the health of your heart and circulation, it is therefore very important that your blood vessels, particularly the arteries, remain flexible and open.

Your Heartbeat

The pumping action of the heart produces your heartbeat, but what makes it happen? The heart muscle, or myocardium, is a unique type of muscle which functions without any outside stimulus. Electrical impulses which cause it to contract are generated from within by the sinoatrial node, the heart's own pacemaker. This is a cluster of specialized nerve cells situated in the wall of the right atrium. Here is what happens during the three phases (known as the cardiac cycle) which make up a heartbeat:

1) At the start, the heart is relaxed. During this phase, called diastole, blood enters both atria (deoxygenated on the right and oxygenated on the left). The sinoatrial node then begins to emit an electrical impulse.

2) Atrial systole is the second phase, when the atria contract in response to the electrical impulse spreading through their walls, forcing blood through the valves (the tricuspid on the right and the mitral on the left) into the ventricles below. The impulse rapidly reaches another node – the atrioventricular node – located at the crux between all four chambers.

3) The third phase – ventricular systole – is brought about by electrical impulses from the atrioventricular node. These spread through the walls of the ventricles, causing them to contract together strongly. This contraction causes the tricuspid and mitral valves to close and forces blood up through the aortic and pulmonary valves. Afterwards these snap shut as the ventricles relax. Diastole – the first phase – then begins again.

Detecting the Heartbeat

It is the more powerful ventricular contraction that you experience as your heartbeat, and this can easily be felt on the left side of your chest where the apex (the heart's lowest point) is near the surface.

The closing of the valves during each heartbeat makes what are called heart sounds. There are two such sounds, which you can hear by putting an ear to someone's chest. They can be heard very clearly by a doctor using a stethoscope placed over the heart and are usually described as a 'lubb' followed by a 'dupp'. The 'lubb' results from the closure of the tricuspid and mitral valves between the atria and the ventricles; the 'dupp', which is higher-pitched, is the closure of the aortic and pulmonary valves. By listening to these sounds, a doctor can tell whether the valves are functioning properly.

The electrical impulses that co-ordinate the heartbeat, giving the heart its rhythm, can be recorded using an ECG (electrocardiogram) and are seen as a trace on a moving graph or on a screen. In Chapter 4 we shall describe how an ECG is carried out, as it is a means of diagnosing heart disease.

Your Heart Rate

The speed at which your heart beats is called the heart rate. The rate, rhythm (regular or irregular) and strength of your heartbeat can be felt as the pulse. During a physical examination, this is usually checked by a doctor or nurse pressing the artery in your wrist (the radial artery) to feel it expand as blood surges through it, propelled by the pumping action of the heart. It can also be checked by listening with a stethoscope placed over the heart, as described above or, if necessary, by using an ECG.

When you are 'at rest' – sitting or lying down – your heart beats between 60 and 80 times a minute. It beats faster in a child and slightly slower in an older person; if you are a very fit adult who exercises regularly it may also beat slower because it will be stronger and able to pump blood as efficiently with fewer beats. The medical term for a slow resting heart rate is 'bradycardia' (*brady* being Greek for slow). However, a 'resting heart rate' much below 60 in an adult is generally considered abnormal, as is a resting rate above 100, and would need investigation.

During exercise the rate increases, which is normal, and is known as a 'tachycardia' (*tachy* is Greek for fast). This enables the heart to meet the body's greater demand for oxygen and nutrients which the muscles need as energy-producing 'fuel'. Similarly, if you are experiencing emotional stresses such as fear, anger, anxiety or other states of high arousal, the heart rate will increase to prepare the body for action, and this is a normal part of what is called the 'fight or flight' response.

When you take exercise or are under stress, the increased demand made on the heart requires it to pump more blood. This doesn't mean that the overall amount of blood in the body increases: you have on average about 5 litres (8¾ UK pints/10½ US pints) in your circulation, depending on your size. It's the speed of circulation that becomes faster. At rest, the heart pumps about 5 litres of blood a minute, but during strenuous exercise this may rise considerably. A healthy heart can cope because the more the ventricles fill, the more strongly they contract to pump blood during ventricular systole.

Speeding Up and Slowing Down

Your heart rate is controlled by the sinoatrial node (the pacemaker), which is under nervous and chemical influences. Although the nervous system is highly complex and not altogether understood, a simple description can be given of the main ways in which it controls the heart. The part called the autonomic nervous system is concerned with automatic body functions: those we don't consciously control, such as digestion and heart rate. It is divided into the sympathetic and parasympathetic systems. These generally balance each other, but when we exercise or are under stress, the sympathetic system dominates; while during relaxation and sleep, the parasympathetic has more control.

The brainstem – the stalk of nerve tissue linking the brain and spinal cord – contains a group of nerve cells called the cardiac centre. This centre is the part of the autonomic nervous system which controls the action of the sympathetic and parasympathetic systems on the heart. An area of the brain – the hypothalamus – has overall control of the sympathetic system. Situated behind the eyes, it is about the size of an olive. Its role is to co-ordinate the nervous and hormonal systems of the entire body. It also registers our emotions. When, therefore, the signal is received for action, or preparation for action, the hypothalamus activates the sympathetic response via the cardiac centre.

The nerves of the sympathetic system extend from the spinal cord to all the tissues and organs, including the heart. Their response results in the release of two chemicals from the nerve endings into the tissues and organs, and from the adrenal glands (which sit like hats on top of each kidney) into the bloodstream. These are the so-called 'fight or flight' hormones, adrenaline and noradrenaline.

Ready for Action

Hormones have specific effects on their targets in the body, which is why they are sometimes referred to as 'chemical messengers'. The effects of adrenaline and noradrenaline are dramatic. The speed and strength of the heartbeat greatly increases, so blood is pumped at a much higher pressure. The airways widen to allow more oxygen to be inhaled and the breathing rate increases. The blood vessels to the skin and digestive organs are constricted, and those to the muscles, where the blood supply is needed, are widened. Stored nutrients are released from cells to be converted into energy.

When you have finished exercising, or a particular stress has been removed, the body returns to its normal state. Originally, these hormones no doubt prepared us to deal with physical danger – a role they still play when we feel physically threatened. Today, however, much of the stress we experience is psychological and emotional, rather than the result of physical danger. Fighting or running away would not be appropriate responses, but the body still reacts in the same way, preparing us for action. Being constantly under stress can mean that the body remains ready for action. This is thought to contribute to stress-related disorders, such as high blood pressure. Taking regular exercise counteracts the effects of stress, as does learning how to relax. Advice on both is given later.

Blood Pressure

We hear a great deal about 'high blood pressure' (known medically as hypertension) and its damaging effects on the heart and arteries. Many of us are unclear about what it is, and we may wonder whether or not we have it. Chapter 3 explains why it may exist and describes the problems it can cause. Here we shall simply describe what is meant in the first place by blood pressure.

Earlier we referred to the pressure generated when blood is

forced from the heart into the aorta, the main artery (*see page* 7). Each heartbeat sends a pressure wave along the arteries. As already described, the pulse in your wrist is due to the artery in your arm expanding and relaxing as blood surges through it, propelled by the heart. Diastole (relaxation and filling of the heart with blood) alternates rhythmically with systole (contraction of the heart muscle to pump it into circulation). Systole causes the pressure wave when arteries expand, and diastole is responsible for the trough between beats when they relax. It is the systolic and diastolic pressure levels which are measured to determine your blood pressure level.

Pressure not only results from blood being forcefully pumped into the arteries, however. It is also due to the amount of resistance there is in the arteries, which depends on how flexible and open they are. Blood pressure also varies naturally and normally depending on what you are doing and the demands made on your heart. It is of course lower when you are asleep or relaxing than when you are exercising or under stress. Your blood pressure taken 'at rest' indicates whether its level is within acceptable limits.

How Your Blood Pressure Is Taken

Although most of us have had our blood pressure taken at some time, we may not have completely understood what was going on. A doctor or nurse uses a 'sphygmomanometer' (actually a simple instrument) to measure the pressure. An inflatable cuff is placed around your arm above the elbow and filled with air by squeezing a rubber bulb attached. The cuff is tightened until its pressure is higher than the systolic pressure in the artery, and this stops the flow of blood. The air is then slowly released. As blood surges into the artery again it causes a thumping noise at the height of systolic pressure; this is heard through a stethoscope placed on the artery below the cuff. At this point, the pressure in the cuff is the same as the systolic pressure and the reading is taken. As the cuff deflates, the sound from the artery becomes fainter and then disappears, which is when the diastolic pressure is taken.

What Is Normal?

Defining a normal level of blood pressure depends on a number of factors and there is no strict division between normal and high blood pressure. Abnormally low blood pressure – hypotension – is uncommon and results from such drastic things as acute infection, blood loss following an accident or shock after a heart attack. Contrary to popular belief, however, low blood pressure can also be considered normal in a fit and healthy person, and can therefore be an advantage.

Blood pressure readings are expressed as millimetres of mercury (mmHg) because the earliest instruments used a glass column of mercury to record readings. This is still widely used today, although in some later models a spring gauge and dial, or a digital display, may show the readings. In a healthy young woman, for example, a reading of around 120 mmHg systolic and 80 mmHg diastolic – written as 120/80 – would be typical.

It is generally accepted in the 'developed' Western world that the older you are the higher your blood pressure will be. So what level is considered to be high? The World Health Organization defines a blood pressure consistently above 160/95 as being hypertensive.

Simply having their blood pressure taken can be stressful for some people, and this raises the pressure. They may be worried about the result or simply succumb to 'white coat hypertension' – anxiety induced by consulting a doctor about any health matter. Consequently, a diagnosis of high blood pressure is usually not made until at least three separate readings, carried out at intervals, have shown it to be raised.

Lifestyle is undoubtedly an important influence; the more Westernized it is, the more likely high blood pressure is to occur. Since high blood pressure and hardening of the arteries are associated with heart attacks and strokes, the other major killer, there is continual research into how our Westernized lifestyle may contribute to them. In Chapter 7 we look particularly at what you can do to protect yourself.

Natural Protection

As explained in the Introduction, there is evidence that oestrogen, the female hormone which supports fertility before the menopause, provides some natural protection against heart attacks and artery disease during a woman's fertile life. This protection declines at the menopause when oestrogen levels fall. A key area of research now concerns the protective effects of hormone replacement therapy (HRT), which is given to relieve menopausal symptoms due to the loss of oestrogen. Chapters 3 and 7 include the current findings of this research.

The Coronary Arteries

Last, but far from least in importance, are your coronary arteries. They are the most talked-about blood vessels because, unfortunately, heart disease so often refers to problems with them. Their role is crucial in maintaining the healthy action of your heart. The whole heart muscle requires a continuous and plentiful supply of oxygen to function efficiently and meet all the demands made on it. Although half your heart continually pumps oxygenated blood, the heart itself is not nourished from inside, but has its own separate blood supply to every part. This is provided by the coronary arteries and their branches which sub-divide to encircle it like a crown (the meaning of the Latin word *corona*).

There are two coronary arteries – the left and the right – but three may be referred to by doctors because the left one divides into two main branches. These are called the left anterior descending and circumflex arteries. The coronary arteries lead off the aorta just above the heart. When oxygenated blood is pumped from the left ventricle into the aorta, some of it is forced into the coronary arteries. If there is narrowing or blockage anywhere, the consequences can be extremely serious.

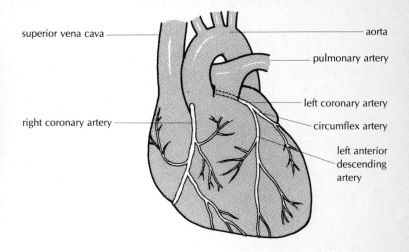

superior vena cava ──────────────── aorta

pulmonary artery

left coronary artery

right coronary artery ──────── circumflex artery

left anterior
descending
artery

Position of the coronary arteries, which branch off the aorta, encircling the heart and supplying the muscle with oxygenated blood.

Since the heart itself in women is generally smaller than in men, so too are the coronary arteries, making them potentially more vulnerable to disease, particularly in women who are past the menopause. The next chapter fully explains the problems which can arise and much of this book is concerned with their prevention and treatment.

Chapter 2

WHAT CAN GO WRONG WITH YOUR HEART

When doctors refer to heart disease, they usually mean its most common form – coronary artery disease. Because women are often not even considered to be at risk, it is especially important for them to know how the disease develops and to be aware of symptoms which could indicate problems. Here we will describe what happens in coronary artery disease.

As previously explained, the coronary arteries provide the heart with the plentiful supply of oxygenated blood it needs to function efficiently. If it does not receive enough blood, its ability to continue driving the cardiovascular system will be impaired. Narrowing and, worse still, blockage in any part of the coronary arteries will inevitably deprive the heart of blood.

The Cause – Atheroma

Narrowing of the arteries is caused by a build-up of a fatty, porridge-like substance called *atheroma* (the Greek word for porridge) in their inner walls, rather like a water-pipe furring up. This accumulation contributes to hardening of the arteries, and is called atherosclerosis.

The process is gradual and can begin quite early in life. Atheroma can be found in the arteries of teenagers – both boys and girls – and is thought to affect virtually all of us as we grow older. This means that the potential for developing coronary artery disease exists widely, as does the risk of other serious problems related to degeneration of the arteries, such as strokes. The medical term for furring-up of the coronary arteries is ischaemic heart disease (*iskhaimos* being the Greek for 'keeping back').

How Atheroma Develops

The build-up of atheroma occurs only in blood vessels where there is high pressure, which is why it is found in arteries and not veins. It affects some areas more than others. Where arteries divide into branches, blood flow is more erratic and turbulent; it is at these points that atheroma is particularly likely to develop.

Arteries consist of three layers: a tough outer sheath (the adventitia) around a strong, thick, elastic, muscular wall (the media), which has an inner protective lining (the endothelium). These three layers surround the central space (the lumen) through which blood flows.

Normally, the inner protective lining is smooth so that blood flows easily, which prevents clotting. The atheromatous process, which may be due partly to ageing and partly to turbulent blood flow at the branches, causes the lining to become roughened. The protectiveness of the lining is therefore reduced and fats in the blood, particularly cholesterol, are deposited there. Fibrous changes in the muscular wall combine with cholesterol to form areas called atheromatous plaques. These grow into the lining and the muscular wall of the artery and bulge out into the lumen.

Because atheroma has a sticky surface, passing blood cells can adhere to it and form clots on the surface. (A blood clot is known medically as a thrombus). These clots may dissolve or gradually become part of the atheroma, contributing to the build-up. The plaques can either steadily enlarge, causing gradual narrowing of the lumen which reduces blood flow, or sudden ruptures can occur in the atheroma, allowing blood to flow into the plaque itself and form clots. These clots become integrated into the atheroma, further increasing its growth. Ruptures may in themselves completely block a coronary artery, which may result in a heart attack or coronary thrombosis, as it is also called (the illustration shows this progression).

The cause of this fatty build-up is not precisely known, but several important risk factors have been identified, and we look at how they relate to women in the next chapter. Although the majority of women who develop heart disease tend to do so from around the late 50s/early 60s onwards, about 10 years later than men, risk factors earlier in a woman's life can influence its development. These factors cannot therefore be safely ignored by younger women, some of whom could be at risk at a younger age anyway.

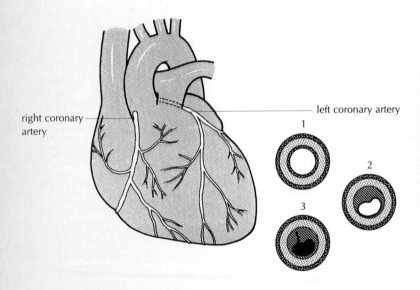

Section through a coronary artery showing (1) a normal artery; (2) an artery narrowed by a build-up of the fatty substance called atheroma; and (3) a complete blockage by a blood clot and atheroma, which can cause a heart attack.

The Effects

In addition to heart disease, atheroma can lead to a variety of problems depending on the degree and location of the narrowing in the arteries. For example, narrowing of the arteries to the legs deprives them of adequate oxygen and nutrients, just like the heart muscle. This condition is called peripheral arterial disease. It causes claudication – pain in the muscles on walking – (after the Roman Emperor Claudius, who was lame).

A weakened arterial wall in the aorta can result in an aneurysm (splitting or ballooning) of the artery which may rupture, possibly with fatal consequences if the problem is not detected and treated early enough. The same problems in the arteries to the brain can lead to a stroke. This is where blood flow is obstructed by a clot (a cerebral thrombosis), or where a weakened arterial wall bursts, causing bleeding (a haemorrhage) into the brain. The resulting damage can impair sensation, movement and other functions controlled by the area of the brain affected. As is well known, strokes can be fatal and are a major cause of death and disability, as is coronary artery disease.

A fragment which breaks off from a clot (an embolus), or a clot itself, can travel via the bloodstream and cause blockages elsewhere. For example, blood clots may form on the lining of the heart after a heart attack and then travel to the brain and block an artery (a cerebral embolus), which is another cause of a stroke. Alternatively, blood clots may originate in a vein in the leg or pelvis (a deep vein thrombosis) and then travel to the lungs causing blockages in the blood flow there. Blood clots in the leg veins can be a risk following heart surgery due to the patient being immobile. This is why activity is encouraged as soon as possible, and special elastic stockings may be worn to improve the circulation (*see Chapter 5*).

Angina

When you consider that the lumen (the central space) in a coronary artery measures no more than about 4 mm (⅙ in) across, and is on average smaller in women than men, you can appreciate how easily it could become narrowed and blocked. The effects of this are as follows.

Initially, atheroma in the coronary arteries causes no symptoms and this may continue even to an advanced stage of narrowing. Why atheroma produces no symptoms in some people is unclear, but this is thought to be as true of as many women as men. On the other hand, it may cause angina. Angina pectoris, as it is correctly known, means pain coming from the heart. The pain occurs because there is an imbalance between the supply of oxygenated blood and the demand for it, so that the heart cannot work efficiently. It's rather like trying to run the car on too low a grade of petrol.

Angina is the heart protesting when physical exertion or emotional stress becomes too great. It is actually more of a discomfort than a sharp, lancing sensation, even though doctors refer to it as pain. Often described as a tightness or pressure, it is like a band squeezing the chest, and can vary from a mild to a severe ache. This usually starts in the centre of the chest, but may often be felt in the throat. It may spread down the arms, principally the left, and up into the jaw and lower teeth, and even through to the back. A severe attack may be accompanied by breathlessness, sweating and, understandably, feelings of fear. The pain usually occurs in the same place, although mild angina is less widely felt.

There are variations in the way angina may be experienced. 'First effort' angina happens with the first real exertion of the day, such as walking up the hill to buy a newspaper or hurrying to catch the bus. It then passes off for the rest of the day. This may be because small blood vessels in the heart, called collaterals, open up to supply an area which isn't getting enough blood.

'Stable angina' is when attacks occur predictably because certain activities demand too much of the heart, which is being deprived of enough oxygenated blood by the narrowing in the artery. If, for example, carrying heavy shopping, vacuuming or climbing a flight of stairs precipitates angina, then it's likely that, on most occasions, these activities will do so again. Over months or years a slow, progressive enlarging of the atheroma could just cause gradual worsening of the angina, so that it still occurs predictably, but with greater frequency and severity. It may become worse in cold weather.

Since atheroma tends to be a progressive problem, another way in which it may become apparent is as 'unstable angina'. Instead of the symptoms being predictable – related to certain types and degrees of exertion – they suddenly start happening for no reason. This type of angina can also occur without any previous warning. Symptoms may be experienced when you are sitting quietly, not exerting your body and heart at all, or they could wake you at night; or angina may come after climbing two steps whereas before you could manage a flight of stairs. This happens when one or more coronary arteries are nearly blocked, or there is a sudden rupture and the vessel(s) may alternately block and reopen again. It is a very serious development which can mean that a heart attack is likely.

Angina, however, can also be asymptomatic – without symptoms. Called 'silent ischaemia', it means that even though the heart is transiently deprived of enough oxygenated blood, nothing is felt. It is estimated that for every episode of angina which causes mild or severe symptoms, there will be another one or two which produce no symptoms. Why this should be so is unknown, but it is evident from ECG (electrocardiogram) recordings that this happens. It is known that diabetes can lead to impairment of the autonomic nervous system and peripheral neuropathy (damage to nerve fibres); this may mean that diabetics with coronary artery disease are more prone to 'painless angina'. Diabetes itself is a major risk factor for heart disease in women (*see the next chapter*). Initially, medication can control the symptoms of angina. In severe cases, surgery or a treatment called angioplasty may be needed (*see Chapter 5*). Lifestyle changes may also improve the problem, and advice is given in the final chapter.

Heart Attack

When a coronary artery becomes completely blocked this usually causes a heart attack. It is often preceded by angina, but can happen without any prior warning. Blockages tend to occur in a main coronary artery, rather than in any of its smaller branches. Therefore all the area of the heart muscle supplied with oxygenated blood by the main artery and its branches could die. This is also known as a myocardial infarction – death of heart muscle. As already mentioned, it is also called a coronary thrombosis, referring to a blood clot (a thrombus) in the coronary artery, or just a 'coronary', which is something of a misnomer.

What does a heart attack feel like? It may be similar to or more severe than angina but last longer. Whereas an attack of angina may go on for a few minutes, or until the activity or stress which brought it on ceases, the pain of a heart attack can last from 30 minutes to several hours. It does not respond to mild painkillers, to the drugs given for angina or to massage, warmth, change of position or any decrease in activity. In fact, the commonest time of day for a heart attack is in the early morning and it may begin during sleep or rest.

In addition to chest pain, someone having a heart attack may perspire, feel cold and clammy, be breathless and suffer from nausea and vomiting. Sometimes the person can faint from the pain, from heart rhythm changes or a fall in blood pressure – or a combination of all three.

Like angina, however, a heart attack may be experienced in various ways. A crushing, vice-like pain across the chest is typical, but pain can be felt elsewhere, as with angina, and chest pain may not even be the dominant sensation. When the heart muscle (or indeed any other muscle) is damaged, a signal is received by the brain which responds via the nerves, producing the sensation of pain. The pain may be felt in the neck, jaw, left shoulder and arm and the stomach, since the nerves supplying these areas are closely related in the brain. Gnawing 'indigestion', for example, can be due to a heart attack if it persists and doesn't respond to antacids or other remedies which previously brought relief. Pain in the lower jaw may be rather like toothache, but may spread across the jaw and down both sides of the neck. Shoulder pain is usually dull, may spread across both shoulders, and occasionally to the right arm, but most often it radiates down the inside of the left arm to the fingertips. Confusingly, it may just be felt in the elbow or wrist. Symptoms such as these can make a heart attack difficult to recognize. They may be attributed to something else, particularly in women.

As with 'silent ischaemia', there is also such a thing as a 'silent' heart attack, which produces no symptoms when it happens, but can leave evidence on an ECG reading. It is reckoned that about a quarter of all heart attacks occur in this way and may only be discovered during a medical check or when some other problem is being investigated. Or there may have been symptoms which went unrecognized by both doctor and patient. Around 20 percent of those who have had a 'silent' heart attack recall feeling that 'something was wrong' at the time when it might have been going on, or in the period leading up to the event.

The Effects

Whether a heart attack is silent or produces symptoms, it can have various consequences. A small heart attack may not have any obvious effects; a larger one can result in 'heart failure'.

The area which was damaged by being deprived of blood forms a scar. Subtle changes in the heart shape can occur, usually associated with enlargement, as a result of the damage. The heart may work less efficiently and the effects can show within days, or sometimes even months or years later. These include breathlessness, which initially occurs on exertion but later may come on with less and less effort until ultimately you're breathless when doing nothing (although not everyone with heart failure progresses to this stage). Fatigue is another associated symptom. Because the heart can no longer pump blood efficiently, the body becomes undernourished which causes lassitude and weight loss. This may not be noticeable since another result is fluid retention (oedema), which makes the tissues swell. It's easy to ignore heart failure in the early stages and put the symptoms down to 'being unfit' or 'getting older', when drug treatment can help the condition.

Angina may follow rather than precede a heart attack. Those who experience it after a 'silent' or unrecognized heart attack may be surprised to learn that they have already had a potentially major problem.

Both narrowing of the arteries and heart attack can destabilize the electrical impulses that co-ordinate the heart rhythm causing cardiac arrhythmia (irregular heart beat). Drugs may restore it to normal and occasionally a pacemaker is required (*see Chapter 5*).

Another consequence of a heart attack can be death from a 'cardiac arrest'. If a severe narrowing or sudden blockage in a coronary artery causes devastating changes to the heart rhythm, the heart can no longer pump blood, the brain is starved of oxygen and this can be fatal within minutes unless the person is resuscitated, as described in Chapter 5.

How the Heart Helps Itself

Just as the body has natural mechanisms which help it fight other diseases, so the heart will try to compensate for coronary artery disease. For instance, when an area of the heart isn't getting enough blood due to a narrowing, blood vessels called collaterals may open up to help supply it, as previously mentioned. Likewise, the body's defence against a blood clot blocking a coronary artery is to break down the clot. Sometimes this is successful and a heart attack is averted, but the process may be so slow that by the time the clot has dispersed, the damage has been done.

Being A Woman

We have indicated that being a woman can help protect you from heart disease prior to the menopause, which is thought to be due to the 'fertility' hormone oestrogen. But we've also said that there are nevertheless risk factors which can make you vulnerable at an earlier age – and which influence the development of heart disease later in life. These risk factors are fully explained in the next chapter. It is still possible, though rare, for heart disease to develop in both younger and older women who are apparently risk-free.

Those women unfortunate enough to develop coronary artery disease still have an advantage over men, however. A study of the Framingham community (the Framingham Heart Study) in the USA, started in 1948, shows that a heart attack is less often the first manifestation of coronary artery disease in women (34 percent versus 50 percent in men). In other words, a woman is more likely to have some prior warning in the form of angina than is a man.

Even so, an initial heart attack in a woman is more likely to be fatal. Women are also more likely to have heart attacks which go unrecognized (about half of which are 'silent'). On the other hand, women do have more chest pain and discomfort which is unrelated to coronary artery disease than do men, and we look at the possible causes in Chapter 4.

Because the symptoms of angina or a heart attack are not always obvious or severe and can mimic other common disorders, women who may be experiencing them could be reluctant to seek medical help, when this is exactly what they should do as soon as possible. Not wanting to 'make a fuss' could lose valuable time, particularly during a heart attack, when professional help is urgently needed.

Many women simply do not see coronary artery disease as being a 'woman's problem' and so may not recognize the importance of their symptoms, and neither may those who are close to them. Unfortunately, this may also be true of some doctors who can be slow to diagnose heart disease at an early stage, particularly in a younger woman. Alternatively, a woman may be aware that she should consult her doctor but fears that 'something serious' will be diagnosed which could disrupt both her life and the lives of those around her. Women frequently feel that they just don't have time right now to worry about being ill. We can only emphasize that looking after your heart is vital, as is ensuring that any symptoms which could indicate heart disease are investigated.

Chapter 3

WHY DOES HEART
DISEASE DEVELOP?

Heart disease is a leading cause of disability and death among women, so every woman should be familiar with the risk factors associated with its development. There is already much advice available and you will probably be aware of the importance of prevention through a 'healthier lifestyle' (*see Chapter 7*).

Because coronary artery disease – the most common form of heart disease – has only recently become recognized as being a major 'women's problem', there is a lack of information on how the risks relate specifically to women. Our purpose here is therefore to explain as far as possible the difference being female can make regarding your susceptibility to heart disease.

Oestrogen

The 'fertility' hormone oestrogen is thought to help protect women from heart disease prior to the menopause, and hormone replacement therapy (HRT) may continue that protection after the menopause, although this has yet to be conclusively proven. It will help in understanding HRT if we explain briefly what oestrogen does.

When a period begins this is the start of a new menstrual cycle. Oestrogen is secreted by the ovaries, a pair of glands the size of walnuts situated on either side of the womb (the uterus). During the first half of the cycle, oestrogen causes the womb lining (the endometrium) to thicken in preparation for a pregnancy. The function of the ovaries is to produce eggs. Ovulation – the release of a ripe egg from an ovary for fertilization – occurs around the middle of the cycle. The ovary then secretes another hormone, progesterone. It 'balances' oestrogen by further preparing the womb lining to receive a fertilized egg and start a pregnancy. If there is no pregnancy, levels of oestrogen and progesterone fall and the womb lining is shed as a period. Another cycle then begins.

At the menopause, which usually occurs between the ages of 45 and 55, fertility and periods cease. The ovaries no longer produce eggs and so oestrogen levels decline. This may be associated with unpleasant menopausal symptoms, such as hot flushes/flashes and night sweats, which affect many women. More seriously, they become vulnerable to osteoporosis. This is a thinning of the bones which can result in fractures and the round-shouldered look seen in some elderly women. Its effects can sometimes be fatal. HRT relieves menopausal symptoms and protects against osteoporosis.

Hormone Replacement Therapy (HRT)

The increase in coronary artery disease in post-menopausal women led to the view that women were naturally protected from the disease during their fertile years. It was also apparent that women who'd had their ovaries removed together with their womb during a hysterectomy prior to the menopause did not share this protection; they had an increased risk of atherosclerosis, just like those past the menopause.

This evidence alone suggested that hormones were implicated. Since the 1960s, when HRT was first prescribed to relieve menopausal symptoms, research has produced evidence that women on HRT reduce their risk of heart disease, possibly by up to 50 percent. Not all researchers are in accord, however. Some consider that there may have been unintentional selection of healthier post-menopausal women for HRT. Nevertheless, the bulk of original studies appeared to show that HRT has beneficial effects on some risk factors for heart disease and does not appear to affect others adversely. Even women who'd already had a heart attack, or suffered from angina, also appeared to reduce their risk of later death from heart disease by using HRT.

Progesterone

Until the late 1970s, HRT replaced oestrogen only, but was found to increase the risk of cancer of the womb (also called uterine or endometrial cancer). Without the balancing effect of progesterone, the womb lining continues to thicken. If this goes on 'unopposed' by progesterone, it may eventually result in unrestricted growth, which is cancer.

Since then, however, HRT has been given 'opposed' by a progesterone-like drug, a progestogen, to women who have not had a hysterectomy. It is no longer considered a significant risk in most women as HRT now re-creates the pattern of the menstrual cycle, though without restoring fertility. The combination of oestrogen with a progestogen is still highly effective in relieving unpleasant menopausal symptoms, as well as protecting against osteoporosis.

When the need for a progestogen was recognized, it was unclear whether its addition would undermine the apparently beneficial effects on the cardiovascular system of giving oestrogen alone. Research into this is ongoing. A recent study carried out in the Uppsala Health Care Region of Sweden showed that fewer HRT users suffered first heart attacks than did those in the general population not taking HRT. This encouraging news should not make us complacent. Even though women are apparently protected from heart disease before the menopause, and HRT may continue the protection, the major risk factors cannot safely be ignored or viewed as less important. Some of them can erode or even eliminate the female advantage.

Risk Factors

As is well known, the major risk factors for coronary artery disease are smoking, high blood pressure and high cholesterol. These can be aggravated by contributory factors such as being very unfit and overweight (obesity), drinking excessive alcohol, having diabetes and – as already emphasized – being past the menopause.

Having a family history of heart disease can be a particularly important factor in women. Those with any close relatives – parents, brothers or sisters – who developed coronary artery disease need to be aware of the greater impact other risk factors could have on themselves. The younger a woman's relatives were when affected, the more her risk increases at an earlier age.

Emotional and psychological stresses can also undermine our health in many ways and can contribute to the risk factors just listed. Consequently, heart disease is often found in those who have several risk factors (it is worth remembering, however, that occasionally it can occur even in women who seem risk-free).

Smoking

Our Westernized lifestyle is an important influence on the development of heart disease. Since smoking is certainly a part of that lifestyle and one of the greatest risk factors, we shall start by looking at how it affects women.

The relationship between smoking and serious ill health is now beyond dispute. Health warnings are printed on cigarette packets, so smokers cannot be unaware of the dangers. Yet the evidence is that women smokers now smoke almost the same number of cigarettes as men, whereas in the 1950s it was half. Although smoking is declining overall in Westernized countries, men are quitting faster than women, and smoking is actually increasing among younger women. Since many of these women are intelligent and know the risks, there have to be some powerful reasons for this trend. In Chapter 7 we consider the psychological and social pressures which may underlie the problem, and advise on ways of quitting.

The Damage Caused

How does cigarette smoke cause damage? According to the British Heart Foundation, carbon monoxide and nicotine are the substances in tobacco smoke that probably affect the heart most.

Nicotine stimulates adrenaline production, which increases the heartbeat, constricts the arteries and raises blood pressure. It is also addictive. Each cigarette is a nicotine 'fix' and smokers are relieving the craving, which is probably why smoking helps them feel relaxed, despite the physical effects.

Carbon monoxide reduces the ability of red blood cells (haemoglobin) to carry oxygen to the heart and the rest of the body. Both substances may thicken the blood and encourage clotting and atheroma. Damaging chemicals called free radicals exist in tobacco smoke (*see page 42*), and other substances in smoke may cause the body to produce more of them, all of which may contribute to smoking-related diseases. The effects of smoking on coronary heart disease risk in women were clearly shown in a six-year study of 100,000 American nurses, 30 percent of whom smoked. There appeared to be no safe level of smoking and the risk increased with the number of cigarettes smoked per day. Light smokers (one to four cigarettes a day) were almost two-and-a-half times more likely to develop angina and have heart attacks than women who never smoked. The risk to those who smoked more than 45 a day was nearly 11 times greater.

The damage caused by smoking is most obvious in healthy young women who have no other risk factors for heart disease. Women smokers undermine the natural protection provided by oestrogen during their fertile years (they may also have difficulty conceiving and can put their children's health at risk). It is estimated that about three-quarters of all heart attacks in women under 50 can be attributed to smoking.

Those who also take the combined contraceptive pill have a 10 times greater risk of heart attacks and strokes, particularly if they are over 35, than non-smokers who don't take the pill. The synthetic oestrogen used in the pill affects the fluidity of the blood and smoking will further encourage clotting and atheroma. Virtually all forms of HRT contain natural oestrogen, which is why it may be protective in non-smokers.

The menopause is liable to start earlier in women smokers, and there is evidence that smoking counteracts the beneficial effects of HRT. Another American study found that there was no significant difference in heart attack rates between heavy smokers on HRT and post-menopausal women not taking HRT. The younger a woman is when she starts smoking, and the longer she continues, the worse the risk becomes. On top of all this, passive smoking (inhaling someone else's smoke) puts non-smokers at risk. Non-smokers with heart and/or lung disease may be further harmed by breathing other people's smoke.

In addition to the effects on the heart, smoking is a very significant cause of disease in the leg arteries, which leads to pain on walking (claudication), a rare condition in non-smokers. Strokes are more common in smokers. It is therefore even more essential for anyone with heart disease, artery disease in the legs, high blood pressure, or who has had a stroke to make every effort to quit.

The link between smoking and lung cancer is well-known. Since the mid-1970s, it has increased by about 60 percent among women, while there has been a 12 percent decrease among men. Chronic bronchitis is also a major hazard.

Smoking reduces the body's immunity (our natural defence against infections and diseases), making us more vulnerable to many disorders. It's worth mentioning cervical cancer here because younger women who smoke are more susceptible to it, as they are to heart disease. This cancer affects the cervix, the entrance to the womb (also called the neck of the womb). Although it is associated with infection by a sexually transmitted virus, cervical cancer is more likely to develop in smokers, possibly because their resistance to the virus is lower.

On average, smokers shorten their lives by about five minutes with each cigarette. The good news, however, is that women who quit may reduce their risk of a heart attack within two or three years to that of women who have never smoked. For those who have already had a heart attack, quitting smoking reduces the risk of having a further heart attack by more than half.

High Blood Pressure

As explained in Chapter 1, blood pressure rises naturally and normally in response to physical exercise and emotional stress (this being part of the 'fight or flight' response). It is when blood pressure 'at rest' is consistently raised that the health of the heart and arteries can be at risk.

We also described how your blood pressure is measured, and indicated the levels generally considered to be acceptable or raised (hypertensive): around 120/80 mmHg is considered normal in a young woman, while a pressure consistently above 160/95 mmHg would be hypertensive at any age. Young women tend to have lower blood pressures than young men. Unfortunately, after about the age of 50, blood pressure in women – particularly black women – rises more steeply than in men, and it also affects a greater number of women.

Although coronary artery disease can develop without high blood pressure (hypertension), and vice versa, it is frequently found in hypertensive people. Again, more women with heart disease also have high blood pressure than men. It therefore appears that with increasing age, women become especially vulnerable to heart disease associated with hypertension. Why this should be so is unclear, but we do know that high blood pressure is related to a number of factors. So what makes it rise?

Essential Hypertension

In the vast majority of people with high blood pressure – both men and women – no underlying disease exists as a cause, even though it is a very common disorder as we grow older. In such cases, it is called 'essential hypertension'. Those with a family history of the problem are more likely to develop it themselves, and this is as true of women as of men, but lifestyle can be a major influence.

We have referred to the 'flight or fight' response which, if prolonged as a result of continual psychological and emotional stress, can contribute to high blood pressure. The stresses in women's lives today that appear to influence heart disease seem to be closely connected with their role in society. We look at these aspects later in this chapter and in Chapter 7.

Our diet is also implicated. It is high in salt, which encourages fluid retention and increases the volume of blood in circulation, so raising the pressure. Hypertension is more common in overweight people (they are about eight times more likely to develop it). Despite the excessive emphasis in our society on being slim, the number of obese women is actually increasing. Unhealthy eating, however, may not be simply a matter of self-indulgence; it too can be related to stress and emotional problems, although other factors – even dieting itself – can play a major part (*see Chapter 7*).

Heavy drinking, which may also have psychological causes, raises blood pressure, although a moderate amount is thought to be beneficial. We have covered the dangers of smoking, which become very great indeed if you already have high blood pressure.

Secondary Hypertension

When there are identifiable causes, high blood pressure is called 'secondary hypertension'. Such causes include certain kidney disorders or an abnormality in hormone production from the adrenal glands, but these problems are unusual and can be easily diagnosed. In a younger woman with hypertension, however, a doctor would probably consider these causes first.

Blood pressure may be raised by certain medications. You should always tell your doctor if you are taking any medication, either prescribed by another doctor or bought at a pharmacy. The synthetic oestrogen in the combined contraceptive pill may, as already mentioned, raise blood pressure in some women. A woman who already has hypertension would be advised to use some other form of contraception. Regrettably, the effects of HRT are sometimes confused with the pill, but since HRT contains natural oestrogen, it may lower blood pressure, in contrast to the pill.

Pregnancy may have a significant effect on blood pressure. It usually falls in the first three months – even in women with hypertension – rises in the later stages and returns to normal after the baby is born. But hyptertension can sometimes be a complication of pregnancy, so blood pressure is monitored throughout. Although in most cases hypertension is transient, in a small minority of women it can persist after childbirth and require treatment. A woman with high blood pressure should be able to have a family, but careful supervision is needed.

The Damage Caused

Untreated high blood pressure can lead to considerable damage. The stress to the lining of the arteries promotes the atheromatous process which causes narrowing and blockage of the coronary arteries.

Persistent hypertension also affects the heart in another dangerous way: it has to work harder to pump the blood, so the heart muscle thickens and enlarges. In some cases, this can cause sudden death because the electrical impulses that co-ordinate the heartbeat can become disorganized, producing a rhythm which is fatal.

In addition, high blood pressure considerably increases the risk of strokes, due to the stress on the arteries to the brain and the greater likelihood of an atheromatous plaque rupturing. Kidney disease can be both a cause and a result of hypertension. Even damage to the eyes can be a consequence, due to weakening of the blood vessels in the retina at the back of the eye.

The main problem, however, is that high blood pressure seldom produces any symptoms until the damage has been done. Severe hypertension may occasionally cause headaches, giddiness and shortness of breath, but most often it is undiscovered until a doctor measures the blood pressure. It is therefore very important to have your blood pressure checked at intervals, particularly if you are on the pill or past the menopause. There is more about this in Chapter 7. Losing weight (if you are overweight) and eating a healthy diet (*see also Chapter 7*) may sometimes be all that is needed to reduce blood pressure, though medication may be required as well.

A variety of medication can be used to lower blood pressure. Diuretics (water tablets), ACE inhibitors, beta-blockers and vasodilators may be given. These also have other uses in the treatment of heart disease and so are described in Chapter 5.

High Cholesterol

Most of us are probably aware that high cholesterol is connected with saturated (mainly animal) fat in our Western diet and that we should all eat less of it. It can help to motivate us if we understand the role cholesterol plays and why too much of it may contribute to heart disease.

Cholesterol is itself a fat (or lipid). It is produced by the liver, mostly from the saturated fat in our diet. Some is absorbed directly from cholesterol-rich foods, such as egg yolks and dairy products, but the total amount of saturated fat eaten is of overall importance. Cholesterol is often described as a 'building block' of the body: it is a component of all our cells.

The level of another lipid, triglyceride, matters too. Also made in the liver from the diet, its role is to provide energy, and any excess is stored as body fat. Several studies suggest that high triglyceride levels (hypertriglyceridaemia) are a significant risk factor in women, whereas most studies do not show this to be the case in men. High levels result from a high-fat diet and, particularly, excessive alcohol.

The overall term used to describe high lipid levels in the blood is hyperlipidaemia.

Lipoproteins

Lipids cannot dissolve directly into the blood and so are transported to their destinations inside minute bubble-like carriers called lipoproteins; that is, they are combined to varying degrees with protein. The proportion of fat to protein is significant in heart disease. Lipoproteins are classified according to their density: the more fat there is, the lower their density. Thus, very low-density lipoproteins (VLDLs) are about 90 percent fat and mainly carry triglicerides; low density lipoproteins (LDLs), which mainly transport cholesterol, are around 80 percent fat; high density lipoproteins (HDLs), on the other hand, are less than 50 percent cholesterol.

The Damage Caused

LDLs carry cholesterol from the liver to the body via the blood-stream. When LDL levels are raised, cholesterol is deposited in the walls of arteries, contributing to the atheromatous process which can be so damaging to the coronary arteries. Here, too, free radicals (*see page 42*) may have a part to play in enabling LDLs to penetrate and lodge in the artery walls. The arteries themselves may suffer free-radical damage, making them more vulnerable to atheromatous plaque formation.

High levels of LDLs and/or VLDLs increase the tendency of blood to clot, which can also lead to the dangerous effects on the heart described in the previous chapter. Conversely, HDLs transport excess cholesterol from the arteries back to the liver where it is converted into bile and used in the digestion of fats. Increased HDLs can therefore be called 'good' and high LDLs and VLDLs 'bad'.

How are women affected? Until the menopause, women generally have lower cholesterol levels than men, although the proportion of 'good' HDLs tends to be higher. At the menopause, there is a sharp rise in 'bad' LDL levels, but there is also an increase in the 'good' HDLs and these generally remain higher than in men. It is the ratio of HDLs to LDLs which is the most important predictor of heart disease, rather than the overall level of cholesterol.

Women's risk of heart disease remains lower than men's, even when their total cholesterol levels are higher. This isn't to say that women with high cholesterol should be less concerned. As total cholesterol levels rise, so do the levels of the 'bad' LDLs, and this tends to be associated with other risk factors, especially obesity. Certainly, lowering cholesterol levels in women who have had a heart attack reduces their risk of having another, and so it is a worthwhile preventive measure for all women.

HRT has been found to lower overall cholesterol and improve the HDL to LDL ratio after the menopause. It can sometimes raise triglyceride levels, although this depends on the form in which it is given. Taken orally as a daily pill, the oestrogen in HRT affects the secretion of VLDLs from the liver and so increases triglycerides. When given via a skin patch, implant under the skin or vaginal cream/tablet, the oestrogen does not pass through the digestive system; trigliceride levels may then remain the same or be reduced. It is therefore inadvisable for women with hyper-triglyceridaemia to take oral HRT.

Cholesterol Levels

How do you know if you have high cholesterol? The answer is that you don't. Like high blood pressure, high cholesterol may run in families, and a family history of heart attacks in early middle age suggests this possibilty.

About one in 500 people have familial hypercholesterolaemia, more simply known as FH, which is genetic (inherited) and present from birth. Far more commonly, however, a raised cholesterol level is not due to an inherited genetic factor.

If cholesterol levels are high, yellowish deposits (called *xanthelasmatha*, the Greek for yellow) may develop on the eyelids. *Arcus senilis*, a fine white fatty ring around the outer rim of the iris – the coloured part of the eye – can be another indication, although it is also a natural sign of ageing.

The only reliable way to measure lipids is from a blood sample, which a doctor removes by syringe from a vein in your arm (*see Chapter 4*). Measurements are expresssed as millimoles – concentrations of lipids – per litre (mmol/l), though it isn't necessary to take a litre of blood to work this out!

With increasing age, women generally have higher lipid levels than men, but because the proportion of 'good' HDLs rises, it is difficult to issue guidelines as to what constitutes a 'normal' cholesterol level in women. Earlier guidelines were based on research in men and made no distinction between the sexes. These suggested that women with a cholesterol level above 6.5 mmol/l required medical advice on lowering lipids. This would have resulted in the vast majority of women aged over 55 needing such advice. There were many criticisms of this approach, and it is now recognized that raised lipid levels should be considered together with any risk factors for heart disease that an individual woman may have, rather than being measured and assessed in isolation.

A woman with raised lipid levels and other risk factors would be advised to make the necessary lifestyle changes, such as adopting a low-fat diet, reducing her alcohol intake, losing weight and taking more exercise (as described in the last chapter). If she is pre-menopausal, she should not take the combined pill, as it has an adverse effect on lipids, again due to the synthetic oestrogen. She certainly should not smoke. Such changes in lifestyle may be enough to raise the proportion of HDLs and lower the overall level of lipids. Medication may be needed if these measures fail to improve the 'lipid profile' (as it is described by doctors). Those with FH nearly always require treatment, however.

Diabetes

In women, diabetes is strongly associated with coronary artery disease and more than doubles their risk. It also appears to be a greater risk factor than for men. The female advantage is lost and the risk exceeds even that of smoking. Researchers are particularly interested in why Asians, both women and men, living in Western society have a high incidence of heart disease and diabetes. Mexican-Americans are also at increased risk compared to Americans of European origin.

Diabetes mellitus, as it is correctly called, is a disorder affecting the body's ability to utilize glucose, a simple form of sugar. Glucose is derived from carbohydrates in the diet (starches and sugars, found in vegetables, cereals, fruit and in many food products – *see Chapter 7*). It provides the instant supply of energy needed to maintain all the body's processes, known as metabolism. Any glucose which isn't used is converted into glycogen (a form of starch) and fat for storage. When more energy is required, glycogen is converted back into glucose for use.

The pancreas, a gland located behind the stomach, secretes the hormone insulin which is responsible for the absorption of glucose for use by cells or for storage. Diabetes results when there is either too little insulin or the body becomes resistant to its actions, causing levels of glucose in the blood to become abnormally high (hyperglycaemia). This is detected from samples of blood and urine. A normal level of glucose is around 5 mmol/l, but higher levels may indicate diabetes.

There are two kinds of diabetes. The first, called Type 1 or insulin-dependent diabetes, usually first appears in children or young adults and develops rapidly. Daily injections of insulin are needed to control the level of glucose in the bloodstream. The second, Type 2 or non-insulin-dependent diabetes, develops more gradually and is relatively common. It generally affects older people and is associated with obesity. With this type, some insulin is produced, but the body is resistant to its actions.

In many cases, Type 2 diabetes is latent (hidden) and only detected during a routine check. An improved diet and weight loss may be enough to establish normal glucose levels, though medication in tablet form can be needed. Diabetes can also develop during pregnancy (gestational diabetes). It usually disappears after delivery, but can indicate the likelihood of diabetes developing in the future.

Diabetic women are advised not to take the combined pill because synthetic oestrogen has been shown to have adverse effects on the way the body utilizes carbohydrates. HRT, on the other hand, may have a beneficial effect on glucose and insulin levels.

The Damage Caused

It is not really known how diabetes predisposes people – particularly women – to atheroma. However, diabetics frequently have other risk factors associated with coronary artery disease, such as obesity, high blood pressure and high lipids. Probably all these factors act together to increase the risk of damage to the coronary arteries.

Contributory Factors

We have indicated how obesity, excessive alcohol and stress can contribute to the risk factors for heart disease. In Chapter 7 we will be considering what can be done to help resolve these problems. There are, however, some points that should be made here.

Obesity

How exactly is obesity defined? Weight must be related to height to determine obesity. Body mass index (BMI) is the method most often used to define it. You can work this out for yourself, but it helps to have a calculator. You take your height measurement, then square it (multiply it by itself); you then divide your weight by the answer. This gives you your BMI. For example, if your height is 1.63 m (5 ft 4 in) and you weigh 63 kg (139 lb), the calculation in metric units is 1.63 x 1.63 giving 2.66. Now divide your weight – 63 kg – by this figure and the answer is 23.68, your BMI.

The risks associated with heart disease increase considerably if the BMI exceeds about 28, and a BMI of over 30 is definitely obese. Weight reduction is certainly necessary, but a doctor needs to be consulted first. *(See the chart in Chapter 7 which gives acceptable weight ranges for women.)*

In the Framingham Heart Study, the risk of developing cardiovascular disease was shown to be 10 times greater in obese women. It is not only the amount of weight which can be significant, however, it is also the distribution of fat. Prior to the menopause, it is natural for women of normal weight to carry more fat on their hips than men. Post-menopausally, this tends to redistribute to the waist and stomach, which is where men have more fat. (Interestingly, HRT seems to redistribute the fat to the hips.) In obese women the distribution of fat becomes the same as in obese men. This is associated with high blood pressure, diabetes and coronary heart disease in both sexes.

Excessive Alcohol

In addition to its adverse effects on lipids, excess alcohol can directly damage the heart. Heavy drinking over several years can be toxic (poisonous) to the heart muscle so that it enlarges and heart failure develops, as described in the previous chapter. Because heavy drinkers tend not to eat sensibly, vitamin deficiencies can result, which also predispose to heart failure.

Recovery is possible if drinking is stopped and diet improved.

If, however, smoking and excess alcohol are combined, the risk of heart disease is substantially increased. Women are currently advised to have no more than a couple of small glasses of alcohol a day (no more than 14 a week), and not on an empty stomach. At this moderate level, it may even benefit the heart by lowering lipids and reducing insulin resistance.

Stress

Little research has been done into the kinds of stresses which may be associated with heart disease in women compared to those affecting men. Such information as exists holds no surprises. The Framingham Heart Study revealed that working women with children who felt trapped in low-paid jobs had a considerably higher risk of heart attacks than women without these constraints. 'Homemakers' who felt lonely and bored had double the risk, as did those who seldom had holidays. Since smoking, excessive drinking and unhealthy eating are often associated with stress and depression, it is not difficult to see how these factors could interact.

Conversely, another US study of 242 white middle-class women found that those in challenging managerial positions felt more in control of their lives than those who stayed at home. This was reflected in their lower blood pressure, cholesterol and glucose. The conclusion isn't necessarily that high-powered career women always have the advantage over other women when it comes to cardiovascular risk; women are becoming increasingly exposed to the pressures of combining careers with homemaking responsibilities. What seems apparent is that risk is increased in those who feel frustrated or overstressed by their role in life. We look further at these issues in the final chapter.

Free Radicals

Finally, recent research has indicated that chemicals in the body called free radicals, referred to earlier, may cause damage associated with heart and other diseases. It is also thought that they may be responsible for much of the damage to the heart muscle following a heart attack, due to the large numbers which are produced then. They can originate not only within the body but from external sources, such as environmental pollution and tobacco smoke.

What are free radicals? Put simply, our body consists of cells which are made up of molecules, each of which has pairs of electrons. The pairing is important to our health. Free radicals have unpaired electrons which can attack other molecules and cause cell damage.

Oxygen is required by the body for processes which release energy (called oxidation), during which small numbers of free radicals are produced. But there are also protective mechanisms in the form of free-radical scavengers which exist to prevent damage. When large numbers of free radicals are produced, or the body's natural methods of coping with them are inadequate, they can start a damaging chain reaction by converting molecules into more free radicals. Antioxidants, however, are capable of preventing harmful oxidation and 'mopping up' damaging free radicals. A healthy diet contains antioxidant vitamins A, C and E, and substances called flavonoids, which perform this valuable task (*see also Chapter 7*).

Protecting Ourselves

To summarize the message on preventing heart disease: protecting ourselves involves reducing those risk factors in our lives over which we have some control, and finding constructive ways of coping with those we cannot directly influence.

Chapter 4

INVESTIGATING HEART PROBLEMS

'I always thought heart disease affected overweight, middle-aged *men*,' said 48-year-old Anita. 'Because I'm a woman, I didn't think it could possibly be causing the acheing tightness I was getting in my chest as I hurried to work. OK, I smoked and was a bit over-weight myself, but I had my family and a busy job as a packer in a mail-order company to think about, so I just got on with life. That is, until the ache and the pressure started coming on regularly when I did something strenuous, like lifting a heavy parcel at work. It left me breathless and scared, so I went to my doctor.'

Anita's father and uncle had died of heart disease in their 50s and her symptoms were, in fact, typical of 'stable' angina (*see Chapter 2*). On examination she was found to have high blood pres-sure. She was fortunate, however, that her doctor swiftly assessed her risk factors, investigated her symptoms and diagnosed heart disease, despite her being female. Now she has given up smoking, improved her diet and is taking regular, gentle exercise to lose weight; she has also switched to an office job. These lifestyle changes, combined with medication, have greatly improved her health.

Risk factors and symptoms are not always so obvious or typical as Anita's, as we explained earlier. Diagnosis may also be difficult because, in women, chest pain is more often due to causes other than coronary artery disease than it is in men. Nevertheless, it is still essential to tell your doctor about any suspicious symptoms if they persistently recur and interfere with your life.

Other Causes of Chest Pain

So what problems might cause symptoms that mimic coronary artery disease? In many cases, nothing of significance can be found, but the woman must not take this as necessarily meaning that her doctor doesn't believe she has them. The doctor has to decide whether or not the pain is coming from the heart and, if it is, whether the pain is due to angina or some other cardiac cause. She could, for example, be experiencing 'musculoskeletal' pains from the rib cage or the muscles of the chest wall. These could be due to a pulled muscle from exercise which was too vigorous or wrongly performed, or to bruising from a fall or other accident. A prolapsed disc in the spine can have similar causes or be due to the gradual degenerative changes of age; it can put painful pressure on a nerve, resulting in back and chest pain. Osteoarthritis, another degenerative condition of the spine, is common in older people, especially women; it too may produce back and chest pain.

Hiatus hernia is a further possible cause of symptoms that mimic those of coronary artery disease. It occurs when part of the stomach bulges up through the opening in the diaphragm – the sheet of muscle separating the chest from the abdomen – where the swallowing tube (the gullet or oesophagus) joins the stomach. Consequently, the one-way valve between the oesophagus and stomach, which keeps food down, is weakened. Acid and other stomach contents can escape into the oesophagus (called acid reflux), causing the inflammation known as oesophagitis, which is felt as heartburn. Oesophagitis can bring about painful spasms and these can easily be mistaken for angina, and vice versa. Hiatus hernia is very common in overweight, middle-aged women and in those who smoke. Taking antacids, losing weight and giving up smoking may reduce the symptoms. In many cases, oesophageal spasm has no apparent cause, but it too is more common in women. More seriously, lung diseases can cause symptoms similar to angina.

Cardiac Chest Pain

On the other hand, pain may indeed be coming from the heart but not due to coronary artery disease. Chest pain may be related to mitral valve prolapse. This occurs when the heart valve situated between the left atrium and ventricle (the upper and lower heart chambers, described in Chapter 1) becomes floppy. This can be associated with stabbing chest pains, although the exact cause of the pain is uncertain. The problem can run in families and is more common in women, but does not necessarily cause symptoms or need treatment.

A further cause of heart pain is coronary artery spasm. It is rare and the causes are unclear, but again it is more likely to happen in women. As its name suggests, the coronary arteries go into spasm, reducing blood supply to the heart, which produces angina-like pain. This also known as Prinzmetal's or variant angina. Unlike stable angina, which comes on with exercise, variant angina can occur at rest. Pain may happen at the same time of day or night and there may be good and bad spells as the symptoms come and go over time.

Syndrome X is another rare cause of chest pain which is more likely to affect women. The pain may or may not be typical of angina, but the coronary arteries appear normal when investigated by angiography, a technique explained later in this chapter. It is thought that in some cases an abnormality in the function of the small coronary arteries (which cannot be seen by angiography) is responsible for reducing the blood supply through them, causing chest pain at these times. Consequently, the condition is also known as microvascular angina. Why the abnormality occurs is unknown, but those with syndrome X are very unlikely to have heart attacks, nor is their life expectancy reduced by the condition.

Coronary artery spasm and syndrome X can be treated fairly successfully with anti-anginal medication: nitrates to dilate the arteries, calcium antagonists to prevent the spasm and aspirin to reduce the risk of clotting *(see Chapter 5 for more about these medications)*.

There are very rare reports of women developing chest pains at certain times during the menstrual cycle, such as at ovulation and during a period. There are rapid changes in sex hormone levels at these times which may affect the 'tone' in blood vessels, and this could be responsible for the symptoms.

Chest pain also occurs if the pericardium (the protective membrane surrounding the heart) becomes inflamed. Pericarditis, as it is called, has many different causes but the most common is a viral infection.

Whenever possible, treatment of chest pain is aimed at the underlying cause. The more typical the pain is of angina, however, the greater the likelihood that it is due to coronary artery disease. In addition, the doctor would consider whether other problems, including those already mentioned, could be aggravating or masking angina.

Diagnostic Difficulties

There is currently no widely available non-invasive screening test which reveals the state of the coronary arteries, but there are several methods of investigating symptoms. Women are given the same standard non-invasive tests as men. The drawback is that they are less accurate in women and the results must therefore be interpreted with this in mind.

At the time of writing, women are less likely to be extensively investigated than men, possibly because they are perceived as being at much lower risk of coronary heart disease. This means that misdiagnosis is more probable. Hopefully, the situation will change as this major 'female problem' receives greater publicity and is more widely researched.

Women can also help themselves by being aware of risk factors, and being informed about the tests and treatments available, which is where this book can help. They can then take positive action both to protect themselves from heart disease and to ensure that any suspicious symptoms receive medical attention.

If you have worrying symptoms, the information given here

should enable you to communicate more easily with your doctor, who will carry out the initial investigations. Depending on the findings, you may then be referred to a cardiologist (a specialist in heart disease) for more tests and treatment. Doctors and specialists are often perceived as figures of authority; patients can feel overawed and intimidated by them, particularly at a first consultation. But your body is owned by you; their role is to advise you and make the best recommendations, so don't hesitate to ask questions. It is important to feel that you can relax and speak openly about any anxieties.

Your Rights

You have the right to change to another doctor, if you consider it necessary. At a clinic you can ask to see someone else. Similarly, your doctor can refer you to another specialist if you would like more than one opinion.

On the other hand, you are not obliged to have any investigations or treatments at all if you do not want them, but you would need to consider your reasons carefully. As a woman, it may be more a question of ensuring that you actually are adequately investigated and treated.

Reporting Symptoms

In women, angina is usually the first symptom of heart disease, with heart attacks generally occurring later than in men. Angina can become extremely debilitating and a first heart attack in a woman is more likely to be fatal than in a man. Women with suspicious symptoms therefore have every reason to seek medical help.

Were you to visit your doctor because of chest pain, s/he would start by asking detailed questions about your symptoms. For example, what type of pain is it? How long does it last? What brings it on and when does it subside? Do painkillers bring relief? How often does it occur and how severe is it? Does it come on unprovoked, when you are doing nothing? Are you woken by it at night? Have you ever had anything like it before? How much does it disrupt your life?

It can be helpful if you take a partner, relative or friend with you, particularly if s/he is familiar with your symptoms. You may want to do this for reassurance anyway, but another person's description of your symptoms can enable the doctor to gain a clearer picture of them.

If the doctor thinks the pain could be angina, s/he will build up a 'risk factor profile', if this is not already known. The profile would cover the risk factors explained in the previous chapter. You would be asked questions about your family history: whether any relatives have ever had high cholesterol, high blood pressure or heart disease.

Questions about your lifestyle would be very important. The doctor would need to find out whether or not you are a smoker. People are often reluctant to admit that they do smoke because smoking is now almost universally condemned. Doctors find they have to probe quite hard sometimes, so be sensible and, if you smoke, admit it. The doctor would then ask when you started and how many a day you smoke. Smokers tend to be economical with the truth, which again is not in their interests.

Many people say they don't smoke because they gave up when the pain started. The doctor would then ask if they had ever smoked and, if so, the same questions already listed. There are those who say, 'I stopped smoking and a few months later I got chest pain.' This is coincidental, but to them it seems to be the wrong way round, and some even believe that it was quitting that caused the problem!

Other questions about your lifestyle would include how much alcohol you drink, what your diet is like, if you take much exercise, whether you feel under stress. The doctor would want to know if you take, or have ever taken, the combined pill or are on HRT (*see* *Chapter 7*).

Some aspects of your medical history could influence treatment, such as whether you have asthma. This would mean that certain heart medication would be unsuitable. A full history would therefore be taken, if the doctor was unfamiliar with it.

Physical Examination

After the doctor has built up your risk factor profile, a physical examination would follow. The way in which this is carried out can vary. It would focus on the cardiovascular system, but other parts of the body might be examined, depending on what you have told the doctor and how s/he perceives your state of health.

Here is what is likely to happen:

- You would be weighed and have your blood pressure taken.
- If you have high blood pressure, the doctor may examine the back of the eyes (the retina) using a special torch (an ophthalmoscope) and take a specimen of urine to assess kidney function.
- The doctor would also look for yellowish deposits on the eyelids and a fatty rim round the iris, which may indicate high cholesterol.
- A blood sample would be taken to be tested for lipids, glucose and anaemia (iron deficiency). (This involves placing a tight band – a tourniquet – around your upper arm, then removing a small amount of blood by syringe from the vein at the bend in your elbow. Only a slight pinprick should be felt.) You may be asked to fast and not to drink anything other than water for 12 hours beforehand, otherwise lipid levels could be temporarily raised. A morning appointment would therefore be best for this.
- A urine sample may also be required to be tested for glucose and protein (which may be present when there is kidney disease). You could enquire about this in advance, so you will be in the right state to give one, if necessary.
- You need to undress above the waist for the examination and lie on a couch.
- The doctor will probably start by feeling the radial pulse in

both your wrists, to check the regularity and rhythm.

- Listening to your heart through a stethoscope may follow. To assess the heart sounds, the doctor places the stethoscope over different parts of the chest. The normal 'lubb-dupp' noises from the valves are described in Chapter 1. Additional sounds, including heart murmers, are usually due to causes other than coronary artery disease (typically to abnormalities of the valves).

- The doctor would also listen to the lungs for any signs of disease or evidence of fluid build-up in them from the heart, as can happen with heart failure.

- The veins in the neck would be examined, as the blood flow in them gives indirect information on whether the heart is functioning efficiently.

- Listening to the carotid arteries in the neck tells the doctor whether they are furred-up, since narrowing creates an audible turbulence in blood flow. Atheroma here often coexists with coronary artery disease.

- The doctor will feel other arterial pulses: in the groin where the femoral arteries pass down the legs, behind the knees and in the feet (on top of each foot and behind the ankle bone). This is to check for signs of peripheral arterial disease. Pressing the big toenail to see if it changes from pink to white and back again shows whether there is a good blood supply.

The Next Step

What happens next depends on your symptoms and the results of the physical examination. If you had severe pains and, particularly, if they came on while you were resting (unstable angina), you would be referred to a hospital for urgent investigation and treatment as a heart attack might be imminent. Conversely, if there was doubt about the diagnosis, further investigations would also be carried out to establish the precise cause. In some countries, virtually all patients with any chest pain suggestive of heart disease would have further tests.

At the other end of the spectrum, if your symptoms were infrequent or indicated mild 'stable' angina, you might be prescribed medication to relieve the symptoms without further investigation, at least initially (*see Chapter 5*). However, relief from symptoms does not always mean that angina was the cause; the drugs used can sometimes relieve spasm in the oesophagus which can mimic angina. (If the drugs were ineffective, though, further tests would be necessary.)

A diagnosis of angina can have serious repercussions, affecting such matters as your insurance policies (life, travel and health). As misdiagnosis is more likely in a woman, you should be alert to this possibility.

Electrocardiogram (ECG)

Many doctors have the facility to carry out an electrocardiogram (ECG) and may do this routinely because it could be of further help in diagnosis. An ECG records the electrical activity of the heart. It takes only about 10 minutes to carry out.

For a 'resting' ECG you lie flat on the couch. Small tabs, each attached to a wire lead, are applied to the skin with conductive jelly; six span the chest from your right side, down under the left breast, towards the armpit. Leads are also attached to the wrists or the upper arms and the ankles or thighs. The leads are connected to the ECG machine which produces a paper printout of the heart rate and rhythm.

What It Reveals

An ECG can pick up rhythm problems which may or may not be related to coronary artery disease. It could indicate whether the heart was enlarged or working under strain due to high blood pressure, which can be fatal if left untreated.

There could be evidence of an old or recent heart attack which may have gone unrecognized or have been 'silent' (symptomless). Since angina can follow rather than precede a heart attack, this information would be of considerable help in establishing a diagnosis.

A 'resting' ECG would, however, be very unlikely to show whether angina alone was the problem. This is because, unlike a heart attack, angina has to occur during the ECG to register on the printout. The chances of this happening while you are resting are small; angina is most often provoked by activity, unless the narrowing in the coronary arteries is extremely severe.

Referral to a Cardiologist

Beyond this stage you would be referred to a cardiologist at a hospital or clinic. S/he would perform all further investigations and non-surgical treatments. The initial investigations would be confirmed, and a chest X-ray would be taken by a radiographer.

Chest X-ray

Virtually everyone will have had an X-ray of some part of the body at one time or another. It is a means of taking highly accurate pictures of the inside of the body.

For a chest X-ray, you undress to the waist, removing any jewellery because this could produce an unwanted image on the film. After putting on the gown provided, you sit or stand with your back to the X-ray machine and your chest flat against the X-ray film. You then take a deep breath and hold it for a few seconds while the X-ray picture is taken.

What It Reveals

The chest X-ray would show the size and shape of the heart, enabling the cardiologist to check for signs of enlargement which could be due to high blood pressure or heart failure. Abnormalities in the bones or lungs which could cause pain may also be revealed.

If it was considered necessary, you would then be asked to return for other tests. We will now explain those used to investigate coronary artery disease.

Exercise Stress Test

An ECG carried out while you are exercising (also known as a treadmill test) may show whether angina is the likely cause of chest pain, and this is the purpose of an exercise stress test. It will be supervised throughout by a doctor and/or a technician and is extremely safe. The test is stopped if it brings on symptoms. Again, you can take a partner, friend or relative with you, although to ensure that there are no distractions, s/he cannot be present during the actual test. Wear sensible shoes or trainers and comfortable exercise clothes. ECG leads are attached to your chest in similar positions as for a resting ECG, so you need to undress to the waist. A hospital gown will be provided for you to wear during the test.

You then exercise on either a treadmill (moving belt), which has a handrail you can hold, or a stationary bicycle, just as in a gym. You start off slowly, then about every three minutes the speed and incline of the treadmill is increased, or you pedal against a greater load. The whole test takes about 12 minutes, depending on your capabilities and whether or not symptoms occur.

What It Reveals

The cardiologist is interested in the information on the ECG print-out, the amount of exercise you can perform and whether it brings on any pain. If pain and certain ECG changes occur, this makes it more likely that they are due to angina. The level of exercise at which these happen may also indicate how serious the furring up of the coronary arteries could be. For instance, whether you can manage 12 minutes, or have problems after one or two, may give an indication of the severity of the disease.

Drawbacks

Exercise ECGs are of less diagnostic value in women than men, as we indicated earlier. Women have more false positive results.

The reasons for this are unclear, but false positives are less likely to occur in women whose chest pain is typical of angina. An exercise test result, however, is evaluated in the context of the woman's risk factor profile and medical history, not in isolation.

This gives a better indication of how likely the test is to be accurate. Even so, women with a positive result should be investigated further to establish the diagnosis. Those women who are unable to exercise adequately, or at all – due to other health problems, or simply age – also need different investigations.

Thallium Scintigraphy

Combining the results of an exercise stress test with those from a thallium scintigraphy scan can improve the accuracy of diagnosis – and it is suitable for women who cannot exercise. Thallium scintigraphy is similar to an exercise stress test in that it aims to bring on symptoms, but what is happening to the heart is then recorded by camera. It will be fully explained to you beforehand, and the whole procedure is supervised by a radiographer and/or a cardiologist.

The scan is carried out in a hospital X-ray laboratory on a day-patient basis, which means that you are in hospital for a day or less. A partner, relative or friend can come with you but cannot be present during the scan. Altogether, the test takes three to five hours to complete, although you would not be in the lab the whole time.

For the procedure you need to remove jewellery which might interfere with the camera image, undress to the waist and put on a hospital gown. You may be asked to avoid caffeine-containing drinks for 24 hours prior to the scan. Next you lie on a couch which is raised at one end and has pedals like a bicycle at the other. You would then be asked to pedal against an increasing workload. If you were unable to exercise, you would be given a drug which simulates the effects of exercise in the body. This would be infused into a vein in your hand or arm during the test. Some hospitals prefer to use a drug, whatever your exercise capabilities.

When you have exercised to the limit of your capacity (or towards the end of a drug infusion) when there may be symptoms, thallium is injected into your hand or arm. This is a radioactive substance which travels to the heart via the bloodstream. You are then moved under a large 'gamma camera' which rotates around your chest. It scans the heart, picking up the radiation (similar to X-rays) emitted by the thallium. Although the state of the coronary arteries cannot be directly seen, the blood supply (or lack of it) to the heart muscle itself is revealed.

The investigation takes about half an hour to carry out up to this point. Three hours later, however, the scan is repeated with you at rest; the break allows time for the thallium to follow the full distribution of blood within the heart muscle. You do not spend the three hours waiting in the laboratory, but can put on your clothes and relax (don't do anything strenuous). You can eat and drink after the first part of the test.

There are seldom any after-effects, although a few people develop a headache and mild nausea when given the exercise-simulating drug. As only a minute dose of radiation is given, the procedure is considered safe.

What It Reveals
The scan shows if parts of the heart are receiving an inadequate blood supply or have been damaged by a heart attack.

Drawbacks
Although the information obtained from thallium scintigraphy can complement the results of exercise stress testing, there is again a greater likelihood of inaccuracies occurring in women; this is because the breast tissue can mask signals coming from the heart.

The test may be particularly useful, however, for women whose symptoms are not entirely typical of angina yet whose exercise stress test results suggest there may be a problem. Although exercise stress testing and thalliun scintigraphy have their drawbacks, much useful data can still be obtained from them. Furthermore, they are non-invasive and therefore very safe and readily available.

Magnetic Resonance Imaging (MRI)

In the near future, newer investigations may make it possible to look directly at the coronary arteries non-invasively. MRI, for example, is a scanning technique which uses only harmless magnetism and radiofrequency energy waves to produce clear pictures of the heart and coronary arteries. To be scanned, the patient simply lies inside a hollow cylinder in the machine while a computer interprets the images and displays them on a screen. The technique is safe and painless.

Although very useful in many disorders, for cardiac problems MRI is used mostly in research. There is, however, a hopeful development being evaluated in Britain at Royal Brompton National Heart & Lung Hospital. A scanner only a third the size of the huge machines currently in use has been developed and installed inside a touring coach. The aim is to take the technique out into the community so that coronary artery disease can be detected before there are symptoms. Such an approach could become an accessible mass-screening test vital to diagnosis and prevention.

Stress Echocardiography

Although the coronary arteries cannot be viewed directly by stress echocardiography, it can give useful information about the blood supply to the heart muscle during stress. The technique is non-invasive and similar to an ultrasound scan, which many women will have had during pregnancy or in diagnosing gynaecological problems.

It takes up to half an hour to perform and is completely safe and painless. You undress to the waist and lie on a couch on your left side, as this enables the best views of the heart to be obtained. A lubricating jelly is then applied to your chest to ensure that the instrument the doctor uses, called a probe or transducer, has maximum contact with your skin. The transducer is then moved slowly back and forth over your chest to produce images of the heart.

What is happening is that high-frequency sound waves, or echoes (which cannot be heard), are reflected off the heart and translated into images on a video monitor. As with thallium scintigraphy, a drug is infused and the heart is observed to see the effects of the drug on blood flow to different regions of the heart.

What It Reveals

The test reveals the function of the heart muscle. Any areas with an insufficient blood supply, or that are deprived of blood due to coronary artery disease or a heart attack, will squeeze less efficiently, and the extent of the damage is shown. It also reveals whether the heart is enlarged. Echocardiography (*see page 97*) is widely available, but stress echocardiography is used less in Britain than in other European countries and the USA.

Building up a Picture

In assessing the results of these tests in the context of your risk factor profile and medical history, the cardiologist is building up a diagnostic picture. Depending on this, medication may be prescribed to relieve your symptoms and your progress will be reviewed every three to six months or even annually.

Alternatively, a further investigation called coronary angiography may be thought necessary to establish the diagnosis. If medication were to prove ineffective, this investigation could also be the next step in establishing the diagnosis. You would be considered urgently for coronary angiography if you have severe chest pain or unstable angina, as exercise stress testing, thallium scintigraphy and stress echocardiography would be unsuitable.

Coronary Angiography

This invasive procedure is much more accurate than the non-invasive tests just described. Since heart disease is more difficult to diagnose in women, it would seem logical for them to have coronary angiography more frequently.

The fact is that they are much less likely to be investigated by this means than men – not only because they are perceived as being at lower risk, but also because an important reason for the procedure is to evaluate the need for treatment by angioplasty or coronary artery bypass grafting. These treatments are generally considered to be less effective in women, and this may influence the extent to which their chest pain is investigated. Medical thinking is now changing, however, and there is more about this in Chapter 5.

Additionally, coronary angiography is not without risk. Because it is invasive, there is a small chance that a complication may develop as a consequence of the test. Although uncommon, a blockage could occur in a coronary artery during the test and cause a heart attack. Extensive facilities exist to correct any problems. The investigation would therefore be recommended only in cases (whether male or female) where the potential benefit of the test would outweigh this small risk.

If you were having this investigation you would be asked to sign a consent form and make the preparations described in Chapter 5. This is just in case a blockage required emergency treatment by angioplasty or coronary artery bypass grafting.

The Investigation

Coronary angiography (known also as a 'catheter test') can be done on a day-patient basis, although an overnight stay may be necessary, depending on how it is carried out. You would therefore be admitted to a ward or room. The procedure involves inserting a slim, flexible catheter – a hollow tube – into one of the arteries leading to the heart. (It is also referred to as cardiac catherization or coronary arteriography. Doctors might call it a 'cath' or 'angio' for short.) The artery used can be either the brachial artery in the arm or the femoral artery in the groin. If it is the brachial artery, you can generally leave hospital slightly sooner than if the femoral artery is used.

In women, however, the femoral artery is usually preferred, even though it is further from the heart. This is because women's arteries are generally smaller than men's and the femoral artery is the larger of the two (though the brachial artery would have to be used if the femoral artery were furred up by peripheral arterial disease).

Prior to carrying out the procedure via the femoral artery, the groin area needs to be shaved. You can do this for yourself in a hospital bathroom (a razor will be provided). After you have put on a dressing gown and cap, you walk with a nurse to the 'cath lab' (catheter laboratory). There will be at least two nurses present throughout the procedure, plus a cardiac technician, a radiographer and a cardiologist.

The lab is equipped with several large monitoring screens and one or two X-ray cameras. You lie flat on a table which is moved beneath the cameras. ECG stickers are placed on your chest (you wear the gown over them) so that your heart activity can be continuously monitored on one of the screens during the procedure.

You will be conscious throughout, so it helps if you relax as much as possible. Concentrate on relaxing your whole body, as described in Chapter 7. The equipment may seem alarmingly high-tech, but you will be able to see what is happening during the procedure on the screens, which you may find very interesting. As a cardiologist put it, 'We'll talk patients through everything we're doing, so they know what to expect, and we're happy to answer any questions. We do our best to establish a rapport and share a few jokes if possible.' If you are very nervous, however, you can be given a tranquillizing injection into a vein in the hand or arm.

This is how coronary angiography is likely to be performed:

- Sterile drapes are placed over you. Either the area of the groin around the femoral artery or the area around the brachial artery is exposed and cleaned with antiseptic. A local anaesthetic is then injected into one of these sites; this is no more than a pinprick and a slight stinging sensation.
- The procedure is usually carried out from the right side of the body (doctors generally being right-handed). A tiny incision is made with a scalpel into the numbed area and, for procedures via the femoral artery, a slim sheath about 10 cm (4 in) long is then inserted. It has a one-way valve at the end to prevent blood escaping and to secure the catheter. (A sheath is not needed in the brachial artery, as the catheter itself plugs the incision.)
- The catheter, which is no wider than the inside of a ballpoint pen, is then inserted into the artery, but you don't feel anything. It is passed into the aorta under X-ray guidance, and you can watch it on one of the screens.

- When it reaches the openings of the coronary arteries, a small amount of dye, which shows up clearly on an X-ray screen, is injected into them. As it passes through them, you may be asked to breathe in and hold your breath to steady the heart, while a rapid sequence of X-ray pictures is taken (an angiogram). At this point, mild angina may occasionally be experienced briefly. Rarely, the dye can make some people feel a little sick, but this quickly passes off.
- A catheter is inserted via the aorta into the left ventricle (pumping chamber) of the heart. The other end is attached to a pressure monitor. Blood pressure inside the left ventricle at the tip of the catheter is measured. These show up as tracings on the screens. Some patients may be aware of the occasional 'missed beat' during the procedure.
- A larger amount of the same dye is then injected into the left ventricle. You would again be asked to breathe in and hold your breath while the X-ray cameras take moving pictures of the heart (a ventriculogram).
- As the dye passes into the circulation, it causes blood vessels to dilate, bringing on a hot flush for a few seconds. During this, many people feel as if they've passed water or opened their bowels (the effects of the dye on nerve endings), although it hasn't happened. You would be warned about this in advance. There may also be a metallic taste in your mouth for a few seconds.
- If coronary angiography is performed via the brachial artery, the same catheter can usually be used throughout. Three differently shaped catheters are generally needed in sequence via the femoral artery to look at the left and right coronary arteries and the heart. In either case, the investigation takes about half an hour.

Afterwards

If the procedure has been done via the arm, the incision is stitched and you can go home the same day. It may be sore and bruised for a day or two. You must avoid bending the arm or doing anything which might kink or block the artery while it is healing.

Keep the arm straight for three hours immediately afterwards, don't do any housework or lift anything heavy for a couple of days and don't drive for a week. The stitches are removed a week later.

Following coronary angiography via the femoral artery, the incision is deeper and cannot be stitched. After the sheath has been removed, a doctor or nurse will press on the site by hand for about 10 minutes to stop bleeding. You must then lie still for up to six hours, which is why you may have to stay overnight. For the next couple of days you should avoid driving and any strenuous activities. Whichever way the procedure has been done you will need to be accompanied home, as you mustn't carry a suitcase. Ask a partner, relative or friend to take you. The hospital may be able to help arrange transport, if necessary.

Before you leave hospital, your blood pressure and pulse will be checked again. The cardiologist will give you the preliminary results of the investigation and discuss the best course of action for the future.

What It Reveals

Coronary angiography will clearly reveal the state of narrowing and/or blockage in the coronary arteries. It also shows how well the heart is working. The left ventricle may be enlarged, due to high blood pressure or previous damage from a heart attack. There may be scarring which affects the action of the heart. The results of the test will enable your cardiologist to advise you on the appropriate treatment. This might be medication – if it has not already been tried (or, if it has, different medication may be given) – angioplasty or coronary artery bypass grafting. For full information on these treatments, see the next chapter.

Chapter 5

TREATMENTS

This chapter describes how angina, heart attacks and heart failure can be treated. It is important to know the options available for treating angina and, particularly, what to do if you or someone close to you has a heart attack (*see pages 87–92*).

Angina

Medication is always the first line of treatment for angina (together with attention to risk factors for coronary artery disease). Drugs are given which can either improve the blood supply to the heart (vasodilators) or improve the heart's efficiency (beta-blockers).

Beta-blockers

By acting on the sympathetic nervous system, these drugs block the 'fight or flight' hormones, adrenaline and noradrenaline (described in Chapter 1). They can therefore also be used to treat high blood pressure and to reduce the physical symptoms of stress and anxiety.

Adrenaline and noradrenaline increase the heart rate and the strength of the heartbeat in response to exercise or stress. Beta-blockers help prevent angina by damping down these effects on the heart. The work performed by the heart muscle is thus reduced, as is the heart's need for oxygen.

Taken as tablets, this medication is widely prescribed. It is not suitable for asthmatics, in whom it can cause spasm of the bronchi (the airways to the lungs). A calcium antagonist or nitrate drug would be used instead (*see below*).

Vasodilators

Drugs that widen blood vessels (vasodilators) include nitrates and calcium antagonists (also called calcium channel blockers). When the heart has to work harder, due to exercise or stress, the blood flow through the coronary arteries normally increases. If there is a narrowing due to atheroma, the flow may be impeded, resulting in angina. A vasodilator may widen the coronary arteries sufficiently to improve blood flow and so relieve pain. By also opening up other arteries in the body, vasodilators help relieve the workload on the heart, and so can also be used to reduce high blood pressure.

Calcium Antagonists

These drugs work by relaxing, or opening up, the blood vessels in the body. Blood vessel tone is controlled by specialized ('smooth') muscle cells within the vessel wall. For the smooth muscle to contract, and so cause the artery to narrow, the mineral calcium must enter its cells transiently. Calcium antagonists prevent this from happening in the smooth muscle of blood vessel walls, which is why they are also referred to as calcium channel blockers. The arteries are thus opened up. Some calcium antagonists also reduce the force of the heart's contractions and consequently lessen the workload of the heart, which helps prevent angina. Although the calcium which acts on smooth muscle cells is the same as the nutrient obtained from calcium-rich foods, the amount you eat has no direct effect on the heart or blood vessels.

In women, one effect of the female 'fertility' hormone oestrogen is thought to be much the same as from a calcium antagonist. It may help to open up arteries by acting in a similar way.

Given as tablets, calcium antagonists may initially cause

headaches, swollen ankles and flushing, due to the increased blood flow through the tissues. The drop in blood pressure they produce can occasionally cause dizziness on standing up. Any adverse effects generally disappear with continued treatment, although ankle-swelling can persist and, if severe, may necessitate stopping the medication.

Nitrates

Like calcium antagonists, nitrates act on blood vessel walls to relax them. Glyceryl trinitrate (GTN) is one of the nitrates most commonly used in the treatment of angina. It is often given in addition to beta-blockers or calcium antagonists. Fast acting, it is useful both in relieving an acute attack of angina and in preventing it from occurring.

Taken as a tablet placed under the tongue or as a spray directed under the tongue, nitrate medication is rapidly absorbed without having to pass through the digestive system. It is therefore recommended for those who have predictable 'first effort' or 'stable' angina. If taken just before the activity known to bring on pain, it can prevent an attack altogether.

Nitrate medication can also be given as a stick-on skin patch. This is placed on the chest wall and the drug is absorbed through the skin into the bloodstream. The patch is left in place for about 18 hours, but there needs to be a break of six to eight hours between patches, otherwise tolerance builds up and larger doses are needed to produce the same results.

In some people, nitrates cause brief but severe headaches, which prevent them from continuing the medication. For many, however, they are remarkably effective.

Bringing Relief

Many women taking heart medication can continue with normal day-to-day activities virtually free from pain. If they also make lifestyle changes which will benefit the heart, the outlook may considerably improve and further treatment may be unnecessary.

On the other hand, medication may prove ineffective and, as mentioned in Chapter 4, this is when treatment by angioplasty or coronary artery bypass grafting (CABG) may be necessary. Traditionally, these treatments have been seen as being less effective in women, which is a reason why women may be less likely to be referred for coronary angiography.

A brief description of these treatments will help clarify why this situation arose (later in the chapter there is more about how they are carried out). Angioplasty involves a much shorter hospital stay, and recovery is more rapid. A special balloon is inserted into a narrowed or blocked coronary artery. The balloon is then inflated so that the affected part is stretched open. Bypass grafting involves major 'open heart' surgery. As its name indicates, narrowed or blocked arteries are bypassed using healthy blood vessels as grafts. Both treatments can bring virtually complete relief from angina, often for many years, and vastly improve the quality of life.

Changing Medical Attitudes

At the time of writing, medical attitudes to treating women by angioplasty or bypass grafting are changing. Previously, many studies appeared to show that bypass grafting carries greater risks for women – complications and the risk of death at the time of the procedure being more frequent in them than in men. This was thought to be related to gender (being female was in itself considered a risk factor). The smaller size of women's coronary arteries, which makes surgery more difficult, was also implicated. Nevertheless, it was established that the long-term survival of women who make a good recovery is comparable to that of men, which is certainly encouraging.

Recent studies in the USA have indicated that gender is of less importance in itself. They suggest that later referral for investigation and subsequent surgery may play a much more significant part in the poorer short-term results. Women undergoing treatment tend to be older than their male counterparts and likely to have more severe and unstable angina. Risk factors, particularly hypertension and diabetes, are more frequent among women patients and are associated with a poorer outcome.

A study carried out in England at Harefield Hospital showed that diabetes, which is a major risk factor for heart disease in women, can cause more complications during and immediately after surgery. Diabetic heart patients therefore require particular attention to reduce the chances of complications arising. In this study of 482 patients, the women indergoing surgery had significantly higher risk factors (other than smoking) for heart disease than the men, and were on average three years older. Other studies show that, at the time of surgery, women are on average five or six years older than the men having the same operation. Older people are generally more vulnerable to health problems, and so other disorders could also militate against their recovery.

Similarly, angioplasty has seemed to be less worthwhile for women because of gender and difficulties caused by their smaller coronary arteries. These again were thought to account for the poorer short-term results – women having more complications and a higher early mortality than men. It now appears that, as with CABG, important factors in the outcome for women are their older age when treated and their greater incidence of unstable angina and risk factors for coronary artery disease. Women successfully treated, however, have a survival rate comparable to, or better than, men.

Although the short-term risks are higher for women, these procedures are still of tremendous value. Referring more women earlier in the disease process for coronary angiography may be a way of improving the outcome of both treatments for them. Women with severe problems should certainly raise these issues, if necessary, with their doctor or specialist.

Using Waiting Time

If you were referred for either angioplasty or CABG, you would be advised to use any waiting time beforehand to make lifestyle changes (*see Chapters 3 and 7*). These would help give you the best chance of gaining long-term benefits and of making a swift recovery after surgery.

To recap briefly, you would be recommended (if appropriate) to change your diet and lose weight. Being overweight increases the chances of complications following surgery. Above all, if you smoked, you would have to make every effort to quit. Smoking poses particular risks after surgery, which we will explain in due course, and you would not be allowed to smoke in hospital anyway. In addition, some heart specialists are reluctant to perform these treatments on smokers at all because smoking rapidly undermines the benefits. This is a controversial issue, but it does emphasize how strongly convinced experts are of the damage smoking causes.

Some hospitals may offer a 'pre-treatment' session or day, the purpose being to give information and reassurance to patients and their families/carers. It would include advice on maintaining a healthy lifestyle, on the procedure itself and on recovery after-wards. Videos and literature may be available. The heart charities listed in Useful Addresses are also sources of information and help.

Angioplasty

Angioplasty is a simpler and more recently developed treatment than CABG. Known also as balloon angioplasty, or percutaneous transluminal coronary angioplasty (PTCA), it can produce excellent results. The procedure is ideally suited to patients who have a single narrowing not too far down a coronary artery. But it may also be used to help those with severe and extensive problems who are not fit enough for surgery.

You would be in hospital for no more than two days, and possibly for only 24 hours. The procedure is similar in some respects to coronary angiography, although it may take longer to perform. You would be given pre-medication tablets or an injection (called a 'pre-med') about an hour beforehand. This will make you feel sleepy and relaxed, so that any stressful feelings are greatly reduced. Other preparations before the procedure are similar to those for CABG, described later in this chapter, although you do not need a general anaesthetic.

Like coronary angiography, angioplasty is also carried out in a catheter lab (*see the previous chapter*). After a local anaesthetic has been injected into the skin above the femoral artery in the groin, a small hollow sheath is inserted into the artery. This is done by a cardiologist in the same way as for angiography. (Performing the procedure via the brachial artery is occasionally undertaken.) A catheter is passed through the sheath and manoeuvred into the mouth of the coronary artery under X-ray guidance. Then a thin, flexible guide wire is passed through the catheter, also under X-ray guidance, into the coronary artery until it passes through the narrowing or blockage. As with angiography, you don't feel this.

A catheter with a balloon at the tip is then threaded over the guide wire until it reaches the narrowing in the coronary artery. The balloon is inflated – it measures no more than 2–4 mm (⅛ in) – and this stretches the narrowing, pressing the atheroma into the artery wall.

When this happens, some people experience angina, which is transient in many cases; a few may need an injection to ease it. Sometimes nothing at all is felt. The guide wire and catheter, together with the deflated balloon, are withdrawn when treatment is completed. The sheath is left in the groin for a few hours to ensure the procedure has been successful and does not need to be repeated. Rarely, it may be necessary to consider carrying out CABG, for reasons given later.

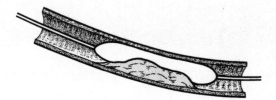

Angioplasty involves inserting a small balloon via a guide wire into a narrowed or blocked coronary artery. It is then inflated, which presses the atheroma into the artery wall. This improves the blood flow and relieves symptoms.

Results

In most patients, angioplasty is very successful. Relief of symptoms is virtually immediate, as blood flow to the heart is improved straight away. Quality of life will usually be excellent and, typically, you will return to normal with few or no drugs. Taking only half an aspirin a day, or a whole one every other day, may be all that is required. This 'thins the blood' and so is helpful for people with coronary artery disease. Aspirin causes indigestion in some people, but an 'enteric coated' kind is available which minimizes this problem. A small minority of people are allergic to aspirin and cannot take it, but it causes few or no problems in the vast majority. Anti-anginal drugs will still be needed if there is disease present in other coronary arteries, but usually in smaller amounts.

Making lifestyle changes is still a vital preventive measure, since the underlying heart disease may cause further problems in the future.

Complications

Although angioplasty is a simple procedure from the patient's point of view, it is technically demanding for the cardiologist.

Complications are uncommon, even in women. Although there is a high success rate, occasionally a narrowed artery may become blocked instead of widened, which may result in a heart attack. In this situation, an immediate CABG operation may be needed, which is why preparations prior to angioplasty are similar to those for CABG (patients are advised of this possibility in advance and are asked to give their written consent to CABG in addition to angioplasty).

Even though the risk of more serious complications, including death, is less in men, the risk to women is still low. Sometimes the procedure does not work, but no harm is done. Surgery may then be required, though not immediately.

The main problem after an apparently successful angioplasty is that the widened arteries can fur up again (restenosis), causing angina to recur. This happens to about one in three to one in four patients, typically within the first six months. Research into why this occurs and how it can be prevented is being carried out at the time of writing. Angioplasty can be repeated, however.

Tiny metal tubes, called stents, can also be inserted into coronary arteries to hold them open. The stent is introduced around the balloon and left in place when the balloon is withdrawn. In particular, stents may be used during repeat angioplasty in an attempt to reduce the risk of restenosis. Their use in first-time angioplasty is currently being researched. Following the insertion of a stent, there is an increased tendency for blood clots to form on it and so anticoagulant (blood-thinning) medication is needed for a variable length of time afterwards. This means that you will have to stay in hospital for a few extra days to be stabilized on these drugs.

Devices other than a balloon which could be used to perform angioplasty are being studied. These include lasers, cutters, drills, suckers and ultrasound. It is likely that the technique will continue to be improved and made even safer and more effective in the future.

Coronary Artery Bypass Grafting (CABG)

Surgery in the form of bypass grafting is the most commonly performed major heart operation and is very effective. In the short term, there is far less likelihood of a repeat operation being necessary than with angioplasty. But it does mean spending about a week in hospital and time convalescing. Most patients recover fully within about three months, although some can take five or six. The length of the convalescent period depends on several factors: the severity of the heart disease, whether there are any other health problems, and on the patient's age (older patients tend to require longer to recover).

Much research is being done comparing the role of angioplasty to surgery in patients who are suitable candidates for both. There is not always a choice, however. Surgery is preferable when there are multiple narrowings. It is also the best option in cases where there is disease in several vessels, associated with damage from a heart attack, which is impairing the function of the left ventricle (pumping chamber) of the heart.

71

Preparation

As with angioplasty patients, those waiting to go into hospital for a CABG operation can benefit from using the time to make lifestyle changes. For smokers, kicking the habit prior to the operation is especially important. Smokers produce more mucus in the bronchi (breathing tubes) of their lungs, and this increases their risk of having breathing problems and pneumonia following surgery. After the operation, patients are required to do breathing exercises and cough up mucus to clear the lungs; this is particularly uncomfortable for smokers. A heart operation can provide the motivation needed to quit for good.

Losing weight prior to surgery also matters because overweight people take longer to heal, increasing the risk of wound infection. In diabetics, healing is slower due to the condition, which is often associated with obesity. Overweight diabetics will therefore certainly benefit by reducing their weight.

There are other hazards related to excess weight. Heavy people are generally less active, so they run a greater risk of blood clots forming in the legs (deep vein thrombosis) and of chest infection after surgery. Your own doctor and the hospital dietician will advise you and encourage you to reduce your weight to a satisfactory level, if necessary (*see also Chapter 7*).

While you are waiting for surgery, you must inform your doctor if there are any changes in your heart symptoms. You must also let hospital staff know at the time of admission if you have a cold or any other ailment that might make surgery inadvisable.

Emotional and Practical Concerns

Little research has been done into the emotional and practical concerns of women facing major heart surgery. It is now more widely appreciated, however, that it is unrealistic and unfair to assume that what has been learnt from studies of men also applies to women. A recent study of women, carried out in Canada by women researchers, contains some helpful information.

The study found that surgery affected the women's innermost being, their sense of 'self'. 'Preserving the self' was vital to them in coping positively with the experience of surgery. The study also revealed that the women's sense of self was very much grounded in two aspects of their lives. One was the ability to carry on their practical activities, their role as homemakers and carers being crucial. The other was the importance of having close, trusting relationships.

Those awaiting admission to hospital over a prolonged period of time struggled to preserve the self. They felt useless and helpless because their heart condition meant that they could no longer fulfil their previous role in life. Women therefore need encouragement from family and close friends to accept that having to relinquish their former role is normal under these circumstances.

When admitted to hospital, trusting in and 'connecting' emotionally with others close to them, or with God, became especially important. Such relationships enhanced their ability to preserve the self during and after cardiac surgery. Successfully preserving the self involved their perceiving the situation as being under control. This could be achieved by their choosing to relinquish control to a trusted person, rather than having a sense of losing control to someone else. Family and/or friends should therefore be closely involved in planning women's care before and after surgery, so that they know what support is needed.

On admission to hospital, some of these women were relieved that surgery would soon be over. They had felt unable to plan for the future and feared they might die. For them, preserving the self was seen in terms of surgery preserving their lives. Others were very frightened, particularly those facing surgery at short notice who had not had time to make any adjustments.

Major surgery is a daunting prospect and a heart operation is undoubtedly a significant life event. But the emphasis should be on *life*. Although the thought that there might be serious risks attached is bound to be frightening, the number of women adversely affected is small compared to those who make a good recovery. The chances of anything untoward happening are not great, particularly in view of changing medical attitudes to treating women earlier. As a rehabilitation nurse said, 'We see patients when they come into hospital before the operation and we try to put any fears into perspective. They stand a far greater chance of life than those whose heart disease goes undetected and who might die at any time. And the purpose of surgery is to give them a better life.'

As we have seen, many women experience chronic ill health as a result of heart disease, with gradually worsening angina, which has increasingly limited their lifestyle. They may be dependent on a partner, adult children or even their own elderly parents. The benefits of surgery can be considerable for them, and their care at home during recovery may be a continuation of what was available before. Sometimes carers are very supportive and certainly do their best to preserve women's sense of self, but long-term ill health can be stressful for everyone involved. Medical social workers attached to hospitals can help patients and their families with any emotional and social difficulties caused, or made worse, by illness. Hopefully, earlier referral of women for treatment will mean less chronic ill health.

A heart attack can happen without warning, however, as can severe angina. In addition to her own fears, a woman suddenly facing surgery who previously led an active life may be concerned about how her partner and family will cope. She may even feel that she doesn't have the right to be ill. If she has a job, she may worry about losing it, as not all employers are sympathetic to serious ill health. She may be anxious about going home after the operation, particularly if she lives alone.

Doctors, nurses and medical social workers are there to respond to your emotional and practical needs, so don't hesitate to ask for help and advice, if necessary. In addition, the hospital may provide informative literature.

Getting Organized

If the practical side of your life is well-organized before you go into hospital, this will relieve you of outside anxieties following the operation. Making the arrangements yourself, if you feel able, may help you to feel in control, but allowing a trusted person to do this for you should also be reassuring. Here are some guidelines as to what may need to be done.

- If necessary, arrangements should be made for the care of any family members and pets while you are in hospital and during recovery, although this depends on how much a partner, relatives, friends or other helpers can do (or are already doing). Your doctor or a medical social worker can usually put you in touch with local services which provide help.

- If you live alone, remember to cancel delivery of milk and newspapers – and lock up your home securely when you go into hospital. It's also wise to arrange for someone to keep an eye on your home in your absence and to do such things as watering plants. Should you feel anxious about your return home, do discuss any worries with your doctor, the hospital nursing staff or a social worker.

- Ensure that you can claim any sickness or other financial benefits due to you. Again, a social worker can advise you of your rights.

- Arrange for transport to the hospital and home again after the operation. The hospital may be able to help with this, particularly if you are admitted at short notice. Try to have someone with you – a partner, relative or friend – especially when leaving hospital.

Admission to Hospital

When you receive notification of your admission to hospital, you will very likely be sent a brochure telling you about the hospital and advising you of what personal items to bring in with you (nightwear and washing things, and other items you may use regularly, such as moisturizer, hand cream, paper tissues, talc and a cologne stick or spray – much the same as you would need in a hotel).

It will also inform you of the services available in hospital (such as radio, television, videos, hospital shops and hairdressing). You may want to take in some books or magazines. If you intend to write letters or cards, take a pen, stationery and stamps. Should you forget any of these, or require additional small personal items and reading material, you will be able to buy them from the ward trolley/cart when it comes round, or from the hospital shops.

You will need to have a small amount of cash with you to pay for purchases and to make phone calls (in a private room there will be a phone by the bed and any calls will be charged to your account). Don't take in large sums of money or valuables, such as jewellery or an expensive watch.

Being in hospital is a good opportunity to sew, knit, embroider or crochet, if you enjoy them. Doing something creative can be a therapeutic way of occupying yourself before the operation and while you recuperate afterwards.

A major operation is a time when we may need comforting reminders which help us feel more secure. Photos of loved ones by the bed and even a small cuddly toy can help (plenty of patients take in a 'good luck' mascot, so there's nothing silly about this). It may be possible for a partner or relative to stay at the hospital the night before surgery, the night of the operation and the following night.

Some hospitals have a chapel or 'quiet room' for use, if needed, by patients, their partner, relatives and visitors. Ministers of religion make regular visits to hospitals, and there is growing acceptance of the differing religious, ethical and cultural attitudes of patients, such as in catering for special dietary requirements.

Voluntary workers also visit hospitals and can be particularly helpful to patients who lack other forms of personal support and help. Sometimes they too have experienced heart problems and so are often very understanding.

Following major heart surgery, you will tire easily. Rest is an important part of recovery in hospital, so be prepared to tell visitors if you are not up to seeing them. The nursing staff may do this for you, or you could make arrangements beforehand for one person to let others know how you are. In a ward where other patients could be disturbed by noise, the number of visitors and the length of visits are likely to be restricted. People certainly should not visit you if they have a cold or any other infection they might pass on. On the positive side, visitors, 'get well' cards and flowers are all good for morale and can help in recovery.

On Arrival

Your letter of admission will tell where to go in the hospital. On arrival, you will be given an identity bracelet to wear; don't take this off until you leave. When in your ward or room, you may be asked to undress and get ready for bed right away as you will be given a thorough examination by a doctor.

Your blood pressure, heart and lungs will be checked. The doctor will be interested in whether or not your heart condition has been stable in the time leading up to the operation. This is to ensure that the reason for your operation has remained unchanged. If this is not the case, a repeat angiography may be necessary. Blood samples will be taken so that your blood group can be checked in case a transfusion is needed during or after the operation. (All donor blood used in transfusions is tested for hepatitis and HIV, the virus associated with causing AIDS.) A chest X-ray and a resting ECG will be carried out so that changes after the operation can be assessed.

Questions will be asked about your medical history, any allergies you may have to drugs, and the medicines you are taking. You will be required to hand over any medications you have brought with you. It is important that you take only the medication given to you during your stay in hospital. If you are on HRT you will probably be able to continue taking it until the time of the operation.

Your surgeon and the anaesthetist will visit you to discuss the operation. The procedure and the risks involved will be explained to you, even though your own doctor may well have done this already. Don't hesitate to ask questions if you want to. You could write down any questions beforehand so you can't forget what it was you meant to ask, and you may find it helpful to have this book with you in hospital.

You will be required to sign a form consenting to the operation (this is a legal requirement before any procedure carried out in hospital). Read this carefully and be certain you understand and agree with what will be done before signing it. You have a right to ask for the consent form to be explained to you, and the hospital has a duty to do this. Even at this late stage, you are not obliged to consent to anything if you decide not to, and you do not have to sign the form. Your treatment can always be discussed further. You also have the right to leave hospital at any time.

The physiotherapist will visit you and teach you the techniques of breathing and coughing which are of great importance after the operation. You may also be visited by a rehabilitation nurse who will talk to you about the operation and encourage you to enrol on a rehabilitation programme to help recovery. An increasing number of hospitals now run these programmes and they are very worthwhile. You can certainly discuss any anxieties you may have about surgery and recovery with members of the nursing staff. You may be able to talk to other patients who have had the operation and are waiting to go home. They can be very supportive and reassuring.

You will have scars from surgery on your chest and leg (where a vein is removed to be used in grafting), but these should gradually fade. At the time when a woman needs this operation, the prospect of relief from pain – and of having an improved quality of life – often outweighs concerns about scarring. Later, however, body image may become more of an issue. Rehabilitation programmes can help women adjust to their new appearance.

If you are in a teaching hospital, you may find that medical students are present when you are seen by a doctor or surgeon and may wish to examine you. Should you prefer students not to be involved, inform the doctor or a nurse. Your decision will not affect your care or treatment. If you feel you can co-operate, you may find it interesting and will have helped to educate the next generation of doctors. Similarly, you may be asked to participate in a research study, which will be fully explained to you, and for which your written consent is required. Again, you are not obliged to participate, and your treatment will in no way be prejudiced if you prefer not to take part.

Before Surgery

In the run-up to the operation, there are preparations to be made which relate directly to surgery.

1) You need to fast for at least six hours before surgery to eliminate any possibility of being sick under the anaesthetic. If your operation is in the morning, you can have supper the night before but nothing from midnight. For an operation in the afternoon, you can have a light early breakfast.

2) Your skin must be as clean as possible to reduce the risk of post-operative infection. You therefore need to take a bath or shower beforehand.

3) Put on the cap and gown provided (the opening goes at the back). No makeup, nail polish or jewellery can be worn, although a special ring you may wish to keep on can be taped over. Any false teeth and contact lenses must be removed. These preparations can be unnerving, but you will be the centre of attention and the nurses will reassure you.

4) An hour or two before the operation, you will be given a 'pre-med' injection or tablets to make you sleepy. When the theatre is ready, you will be lifted onto a trolley and wheeled there by a porter. A nurse will also go with you. On arrival, the anaesthetist will greet you (although you probably won't remember much of this later). You may be given oxygen to breathe through a mask. The anaesthetic is then injected into a vein in the back of your hand and you won't be aware of anything after that.

The Operation

Some patients want detailed information about the operation, perhaps because it gives them a greater sense of control. It will be helpful for them if we describe how the operation is carried out. Others who do not wish to know the details can start reading again at the next heading.

Earlier we explained that the purpose of CABG is to graft healthy blood vessels to the aorta and then to the coronary arteries below the narrowed or blocked areas. A good supply of oxygenated blood is thus restored to the heart and angina is improved or relieved altogether.

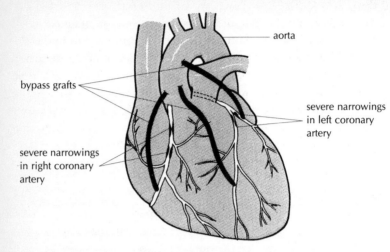

In coronary artery bypass grafting (CABG), lengths of healthy vein, usually taken from the leg, are attached to the aorta and to the coronary arteries below severe narrowings or blockages (artery grafts may occasionally be used). This restores an adequate blood supply to the heart muscle, so relieving angina.

Two surgeons in fact perform the procedure, which can last several hours, depending on how many grafts are needed (usually three or four). The first surgeon opens the chest by making an incision of about 13–15 cm (5–6 in) lengthwise through the sternum (breastbone), which runs from the base of the neck to just above the diaphragm. Meanwhile, the second surgeon makes an incision up the inside of the leg from the ankle and removes a length of vein (this does not have any adverse effects on the leg). Sections are cut from this vein to be used as grafts. The leg incision is then sutured (stitched) together. If the leg veins are not suitable, perhaps due to varicose problems, a length from the arm can be used instead.

To attach the grafts, the heartbeat has to be temporarily stopped and the blood flow diverted. Movement of the lungs must also be suspended during the operation. This is done by attaching the patient to a heart-lung bypass machine (also called a cardiopulmonary bypass or pump oxygenator). The machine takes blood from the body via tubes stitched into the venae cavae, the main veins leading to the heart. Oxygen is then added and carbon dioxide removed. The oxygenated blood is returned via a tube stitched into the aorta, which carries blood to the body, or into the femoral artery in the leg at the groin (although the latter is rarely done). The bypass machine cools the blood and lowers body temperature, reducing the body's oxygen requirements.

Lengths of vein are then sewn to the aorta (using permanent stitching) and to points below the narrowing or blockage in the affected coronary arteries. In recent years, a blood vessel called the internal mammery artery (IMA) has also been used as a graft. There are two of them running inside the chest wall and although both can be grafted, the left is frequently used. The IMA is a branch of one of the main arteries from the aorta, so it is simply a matter of detaching it at one end and sewing it to the coronary artery, as just described. Moving it from its normal position has no ill effects. These arteries, which give excellent long-term results, may be combined with vein grafts.

After bypass grafting is completed, the blood is warmed and returned to the body to raise the temperature. The heart-lung machine is then disconnected. The venae cavae and aorta are repaired where the tubes were inserted so that blood flow to the heart is restored. It usually starts beating again spontaneously in response to the blood flow. Occasionally it is necessary to administer an electric shock to restart the heart. A ventilator then takes over the breathing (this is also called a breathing machine, respirator or life-support system).

Finally, the breastbone is wired or stitched together. The overlying skin is also stitched and covered by a gauze dressing.

Afterwards

Following surgery you will be transferred immediately to the intensive care unit (ICU), which is routine after this operation; it does not mean that something has gone wrong. You will be there for about 24 hours, being looked after by a highly experienced staff.

For around 12 hours you will be kept sedated and remain connected to the ventilator so that your body has less to do.

Breathing

The ventilator is rather like a bellows. It is attached to a tube which passes down your throat into your trachea (windpipe), and oxygen is pumped into your lungs. The natural elasticity of your lungs expels the oxygen and carbon dioxide (a waste product) between each 'breath'. When you come round, the tube will still be in place and so you won't be able to eat, drink or talk. (In the Canadian survey, this was when the women understandably felt least in control; some had strange dreams, due to the drugs given.)

You may be allowed a visit from someone close to you, if you indicate that this is what you would like (you can write down any requests). Although you can't talk, you can hold hands, if you wish, which can be comforting.

The tube will be removed when your breathing is adequate, usually about 12 to18 hours after the operation. While it is there, any fluid which has collected in your lungs is sucked out through it via a thin tube. This is not painful, though it can make you cough. Removing the ventilator tube can be a little uncomfortable, but it takes only a few seconds and at this stage you will still be sleepy. An oxygen mask is then placed over your mouth and nose, which blows moisturized oxygenated air for you to breathe. This may be needed for a day or two.

Equipment and Tubes

You will become aware of being attached to monitoring equipment around your bed and to a number of tubes. It is worth knowing in advance that all this is perfectly normal. The action of your heart is monitored by an ECG. There will be two or three drips into a vein in the side of your neck. (A drip consists of tubing connecting a bag of fluid on a stand by the bed to a hollow needle which is inserted into a vein and taped in place.) Blood transfusions during and after the operation are given via a drip, as is fluid to keep you hydrated since you cannot drink immediately. Painkillers and antibiotics to prevent post-operative infection are also given this way.

There will be an 'arterial line' inserted into an artery in your wrist. This looks like a drip but actually monitors blood pressure. A naso-gastric tube ensures that the stomach remains empty so that there is no risk of being sick while the ventilator tube is in place. At the end of the operation, two or three chest drains (narrow tubes) are placed through the chest wall. These drain fluid from around the organs and help the lungs to reflate naturally by relieving pressure on them. Finally, there will be a catheter (a fine tube) in your urethra to enable you to urinate during and after the operation. (The volume of urine produced is also an indication of how your kidneys are functioning at this time.)

Daily tests will be carried out for the first few days to monitor your condition. Blood samples are taken by syringe to check for anaemia, in case a transfusion is needed, and to assess kidney and lung function. Chest X-rays show whether the chest drains are in the necessary positions, and give information about the heart and lungs.

All the tubes are removed within two days by gently pulling them out, which is virtually painless. People describe removal of the chest drains as a 'strange sensation' but not unpleasant. The stitch which held each of them in place is then tightened to close the small incision, or a plaster is put over it. Only a small scar is left after healing.

Recuperation

After your immediate post-operative recovery in the ICU, you will return to your ward or room to continue recuperating. Many patients are surprisingly cheerful on day two; they are relieved that 'it's over now'. This is often followed by a reaction which makes them feel weepy and depressed. Major surgery is a shock to the system and so mood swings are only to be expected.

Your chest and shoulders will be stiff and sore from surgery, although you should not be in any real pain (but don't hesitate to ask for pain relief, if necessary). The nurses will help you to wash and do your hair. The physiotherapist will spend a lot of time with you in the first few days, encouraging you to carry out the deep breathing and coughing exercises you were taught before the operation to clear your lungs. This will be uncomfortable at first.

You will be out of bed on the second day after surgery. This may seem very soon following a major operation, but it helps prevent blood clots from forming in your legs as a result of being immobile in bed. Wearing special elastic stockings also improves the circulation, and this reduces any swelling which may occur in the leg from which the vein was removed. Mobility certainly aids recovery. The nurses and physiotherapist will help you walk round the bed, then round the room, and will gradually build up the distance. By the time you go home you will be able to climb a flight of stairs without becoming breathless.

You should be drinking again on the second day, and should try to eat something light, even though you may not feel like it. The digestive system tends to shut down because of the anaesthetic, and so you may have indigestion and wind to start with. The nurses can give you remedies, if necessary.

Before you leave hospital your stitches will be removed by a nurse (unless soluble ones were used, which will simply dissolve away). Removal does not hurt if done gently. It is not unusual for a little fluid or blood to leak from the incisions in the chest and leg. A dry dressing is all that is needed. You will be given a thorough check by a doctor and, if all test results are satisfactory, you can then go home. In Chapter 6 we will advise on recovery and rehabilitation after leaving hospital.

Results

In the majority of CABG patients, angina is completely relieved and in a minority, it is much improved. Because activity is no longer limited by severe pain and the heart has a better blood supply, you may become as active again as you were before having angina. Brisk walking, jogging and playing tennis may all be possible, and indeed are good for the heart and circulation, although exercise which involves weight training is not advisable (there is more about exercise in the next two chapters).

When fully recovered, you are usually fit enough to go back to work, if you have a job outside the home. It is in fact beneficial to resume as much of your former life as you can. Half an aspirin a day or a whole one every other day, as after angioplasty, is generally the only medication needed (an enteric-coated kind will prevent indigestion). Occasionally, medication to stablize the heart rhythm may be initially required.

Taking diuretics (water tablets) may be necessary for a few weeks post-operatively; the heart muscle has to recover and so fluid may build up in the lungs, which needs to be removed. (Diuretics remove excess water and salt from the body by increasing the amount lost in urine. This also has the effect of lowering blood pressure, and so diuretics are used in the treatment of hypertension.)

Neither bypass surgery nor angioplasty can, however, repair a heart which has been damaged by a heart attack. But by relieving pain, they permit the person to have the best quality of life possible. Neither do these treatments cure the underlying heart disease. The atheromatous process can continue and cause problems in the future, which is why lifestyle changes remain so important after both procedures.

Complications

Before the operation you will be advised of complications that might occur at the time of the procedure or shortly afterwards. Do not be alarmed, as they are potential rather than probable. Serious complications – a heart attack or stroke – may arise both from the stresses of the procedure and the condition of the patient. Heart disease is often accompanied by furring up of other arteries. When those to the brain are affected, a stroke during or after surgery is a possibility. These serious complications become much less likely a day or two later.

The heart rhythm is usually normal following surgery, but occasionally atrial fibrillation can develop soon afterwards: the atria (the upper chambers of the heart) beat much faster than the ventricles (the lower chambers). This erratic heartbeat can be corrected by medication, or by applying an electric shock via defibrillator paddles placed on the chest over the heart. The latter procedure is performed under a short-acting general anaesthetic so that nothing is felt.

There is the possibility of a chest infection, which can be treated with antibiotics. Wound infection may occur, particularly in diabetics, for the reasons given earlier. The bacteria that cause the infection exist on our skin and in the air around us. Wound infection can also be treated with antibiotics.

If you experience any of the following after returning home, contact your doctor or the hospital: severe palpitations, severe breathlessness, chest pain, fever and sweating, severe dizziness or disturbances in vision. These reactions do not necessarily mean that anything has gone wrong with your heart, but you should have them checked out.

In the longer term, it is possible for vein grafts to fur up, causing angina to recur. The furring up is due to atheroma, since veins themselves are not ideally suited to being in a high-pressure arterial system. As a result, changes can gradually take place in their structure which cause them to narrow (there is much research being carried out into why these problems occur).

The use of the IMA graft has long-term advantages because it is an artery and not a vein. It is not always possible to use the IMA, however, and this is more often true in diabetic women where its quality may not be so good. Sometimes it is too small anyway. There is increasing interest among cardiac surgeons – particularly in France – in using the radial artery in the forearm because it may have better long-term results. Similarly, using the gastroepiploic artery, which supplies part of the stomach, is another possibility.

Should severe angina recur due to a narrowed graft, a repeat bypass operation can be carried out. Alternatively, it may be possible to use angioplasty to widen the graft and, if necessary, to insert stents to hold it open, so avoiding another big operation.(Angiography will show which treatment is appropriate.) Sometimes repeat surgery is not an option, due to the patient's health. In such cases, angioplasty may bring about improvements.

Heart Attack

In Chapter 2 we explained what happens during a heart attack and how to recognize the symptoms. Everyone should be aware of these facts, not only because we might suffer from a heart attack one day, but also because we might be with someone who has a heart attack. We should also, therefore, know what to do in either of these situations to ensure that expert medical treatment is received *without delay*. A suspected heart attack should *always* be treated as an emergency.

To summarize the information given earlier, a heart attack occurs when a coronary artery becomes blocked and the heart muscle in that area is damaged through being deprived of oxygenated blood. Typically, this causes a crushing, vice-like pain across the chest, which can last for 30 minutes or longer – unlike angina, which is less prolonged. The pain may radiate up into the jaw, through to the back or across the shoulders and, usually, down the left arm; it may also be felt in the stomach region. Sometimes it occurs in only one of these places. Mild painkillers and other home remedies do not work. In addition, the person may perspire and feel cold and clammy; breathlessness and nausea may follow. Fainting may result from severe pain, changes in heart rhythm or a fall in blood pressure, or a combination of all three.

Although angina is usually the first symptom of heart disease in women, a heart attack can still occur unexpectedly without previous angina. It is therefore important to be alert to this possibility, and not to assume that symptoms which could indicate a heart attack must be due to something else in a woman. Even an apparently 'mild' heart attack can sometimes have serious consequences, so it is essential to take any suspicious symptoms seriously.

In the event of a suspected heart attack, there are two courses of action to be taken immediately.

1) The first is to summon medical help. Call the doctor, who can give advice and, if necessary, may be able to provide help faster than an ambulance. If not, call an ambulance. Speedy

action is essential since 60 percent of deaths from heart attacks occur within the first hour from the onset of pain. The woman should sit back in a chair while waiting, as this makes breathing easier. If she is very near a hospital when the suspected attack happens, the best course of action may be for someone to drive her there directly.

2) The second is for her to chew on a plain, uncoated aspirin – if she is conscious – because of its anti-clotting action. It is more quickly absorbed if chewed. (Do not confuse aspirin with other painkillers which have no value in treating a heart attack.) This is preferable to soluble aspirin, which has to be dissolved in water. Ideally, fluids should not be taken because of the risk of inhaling stomach contents should fainting occur. If only soluble aspirin is available, however, it is better to take it than not.

Cardiac Arrest

If the woman collapses and loses consciousness, it is vital to establish whether she has simply fainted or suffered a cardiac arrest. The latter is where a heart attack causes devastating changes to the heart rhythm so that effective pumping ceases. The disturbance to the electrical impulses controlling the heart rhythm can result in ventricular fibrillation, where the lower pumping chambers twitch rapidly in a completely disorganized manner. Consequently, the supply of blood to the brain (and the rest of the body) is interrupted and if this is not restored, brain damage or death can occur within minutes.

Immediate action must be taken by anyone present. If you do not have first aid training and others are there, start by asking if someone has this training. If no one has, then the simple emergency procedures given next can be carried out by anybody.

1) *Establish whether the woman is unconscious.* Gently shake her and say loudly, 'Can you hear me?'. If there is no response and you are alone, shout for help. Then swiftly assess as follows.

2) *Open the airway.* Kneel beside the woman and open the airway

by tilting her head back, lifting her chin and opening her mouth.

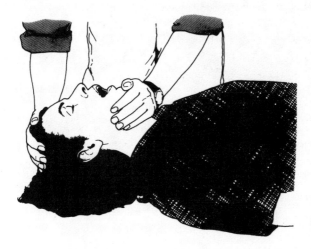

3) *Check for breathing.* Look, listen and feel for signs of breathing. If she is still breathing, then a cardiac arrest is unlikely.
4) *Feel the pulse in the neck.* Place two fingers on her neck below the chin and slide them into the natural hollow at the side of the neck where the carotid artery pulse is located.

If she is not breathing and has no pulse, call for an ambulance. Then you must start cardiopulmonary resuscitation straight away.

Cardiopulmonary Resuscitation (CPR)

This procedure can restore a temporary supply of blood until medical help arrives. It combines mouth-to-mouth ventilation with chest compression. You must do the following:

1) Place her on the floor, face upwards.
2) *Clear the airway,* as before, by tilting her head back, lifting her chin and opening her mouth.
3) *Give two breaths.* Pinch her nostrils between your finger and thumb and place your lips around her mouth. Blow into the

mouth until her chest rises. Let it fall before giving the second breath.

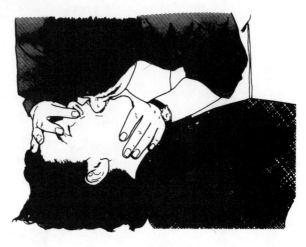

4) *Compress the chest 15 times in quick succession.* First, feel for the lower end of the breastbone, then measure two finger widths above this. Place the heel of one hand on the breastbone at this point and put the other hand on top. Lean over the woman, keeping your arms straight, and press down firmly but smoothly 15 times, giving slightly more than one compression per second.

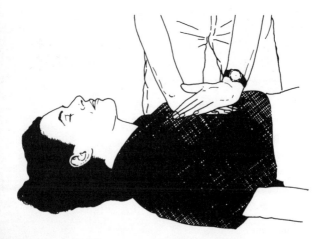

5) *Repeat two breaths, then 15 compressions, until medical help arrives.* CPR can be tiring, so if you need a break, ask someone else to take over, if possible. Two people can perform CPR, one giving mouth-to-mouth ventilation and the other chest compression. In this situation, one breath should be given for every five compressions.

6) If a pulse is present but the woman is not breathing, give 10 breaths without compressions. Call an ambulance if there is no response, then reassess the woman's condition.

7) *Definitely do not start CPR if the woman has simply fainted.* This can cause further harm during a heart attack. Place her in the 'recovery position' (roll her gently onto her side facing you; bend the uppermost arm and leg to support her body and to prevent her from rolling onto her face; tilt her head back and open her mouth to clear the airway). Cover her with a blanket or coat, if available, and stay with her until medical help arrives.

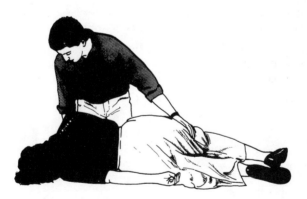

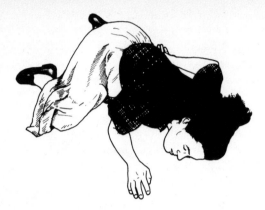

8) *Never try out CPR on a conscious person as a way of learning the technique.* Attend a training session, as advised next, where you will be able to practise on a resuscitation manikin.

Public Awareness

Heart charities are striving towards enabling everyone to recognize a heart attack or cardiac arrest – and to know what action they should take. Sadly, many people delay calling medical help because they just don't recognize the symptoms, or they may dismiss their significance in a woman because of the still widely held belief that 'only men have heart attacks'.

Even when someone has collapsed, most people still have little or no idea of the immediate action required. Many lives could be saved if emergency aid was given right away. Heart charities are encouraging emergency aid training in schools and the community; you can learn the basics in a simple two-hour session. Taking refresher sessions is also recommended, as is carrying a small CPR instruction card with you at all times. See Useful Addresses for organizations you can contact for information on emergency aid training.

Medical Treatments

How is a heart attack or cardiac arrest treated medically? We will continue by describing first how a victim of a cardiac arrest is helped.

Treating Cardiac Arrest

The emergency ambulance crew will continue CPR. Most hospitals have a cardiac arrest team on standby, so when the ambulance arrives at the hospital, CPR can be taken over immediately by the staff. Some ambulances are equipped with a defibrillator, which can deliver an electric shock to correct certain abnormal heart rhythms, such as ventricular fibrillation.

The patient is taken into the resuscitation room and, if her condition stabilizes, she will go into intensive care or into a coronary care unit (CCU) dedicated to heart problems. If necessary, she will be put on a ventilator and be given strong supporting drugs intravenously. There is a high risk of brain damage or death following a cardiac arrest, so prompt action in the first place is essential.

Treating a Heart Attack

In the case of a heart attack, we have already stressed the importance of getting to a hospital as fast as possible. Thrombolytic drugs (the so-called 'clot-busters') need to be given intravenously to dissolve the blood clot in the coronary artery which has caused the heart attack. The sooner these drugs are administered, the greater the benefit. The aim is to prevent irreversible damage to the heart muscle, if possible. After about 12 hours, these drugs are of very little benefit. Research is being carried out into the possibility of family doctors carrying them so they could be given much earlier, when the patient is still at home.

Emergency ambulance crews have the expertise and equipment needed to stabilize the patient's condition as much as possible before and during the journey to hospital. A woman having a heart attack would be given oxygen to breathe through a mask. She may be given a drip into a vein in her hand or forearm, to establish access for medication given in hospital, and her heart rate and rhythm would be monitored by ECG to show whether pain was coming from the heart and to provide a record for the hospital. Any serious changes in heart rhythm would register on the ECG and appropriate action could therefore be taken.

In hospital, she would usually be treated in a CCU. The diagnosis of a heart attack is confirmed from the woman's account of her symptoms, from an ECG recording and from blood tests to measure specific enzymes (proteins) released into the bloodstream from damaged heart muscle cells.

Medication

The 'clot-buster' drugs already mentioned are rapidly given, either as a one-off injection or via an intravenous infusion over several minutes or hours, depending on the drug used. These include streptokinase, anistreplase and tissue plasminogen activator (tPA). They all act by increasing the levels of a substance in the blood called plasmin which dissolves clots. Pain relief is administered as required and aspirin is given.

Depending on the severity of the heart attack, other drugs may be given. Beta-blockers, described earlier, can help prevent abnormal rhythm changes. Angiotensin converting enzyme (ACE) inhibitors help the heart muscle to recover. Taken by mouth, ACE inhibitors prevent, or inhibit, a substance in the blood called angiotensin I from being converted into an active form (angiotensin II) which constricts blood vessels and raises blood pressure. They thus have the opposite effect, and so are often also used together with diuretics in the treatment of high blood pressure and heart failure.

Following a heart attack, a woman would continue taking aspirin for life (half a tablet each day or a whole one every other day), as after angioplasty or CABG. Beta-blockers and ACE inhibitors may be continued for a variable length of time.

Abnormal Heart Rhythms

Following a heart attack, the heart rhythm may change to produce abnormally slow or fast rhythms. Many abnormal heart rhythms are short-lived and settle down soon after a heart attack as the heart heals and recovers. Rarely, problems with heart rhythm persist. Very severe fast or slow rhythms may cause loss of consciousness.

Very slow rhythms may require a pacemaker. This may be needed for only a few days until the rhythm returns to normal, or as a permanent device. A fine, flexible lead is passed to the heart, under X-ray guidance, via a vein in the neck (only a local anesthetic is necessary). The lead is then attached to the pacemaker. This small device contains special batteries which emit electrical impulses and take over the heart rhythm if it slows below a safe level. A temporary external pacemaker can be placed on a bedside cabinet or worn on a belt. If a permanent pacemaker is required, it is inserted under the skin, just below the collarbone, which leaves a small scar. Implantation is done under local anaesthetic.

Medication may control fast rhythms, but if these continue despite treatment, an investigation called an electrophysiological study (EPS) may be carried out.

From the patient's point of view, this procedure is similar in some respects to coronary angiography (*see pages 58–62*) since it involves the insertion of catheters into the heart via blood vessels in the groin and elsewhere. The purpose, however, is to test the conduction of electrical impulses in the heart, and it may also be used to treat the abnormal rhythm.

More recently, a miniaturized implantable defibrillator, similar to a pacemaker, has been designed which can deliver small electric shocks to the heart. If the rhythm becomes abnormally fast, the defibrillator can be used to restore a normal heartbeat. Patients with severely fast rhythms which do not respond to conventional treatments are potential candidates for this device.

Further Treatment

If a woman with a heart attack were admitted to a centre with facilities for angiography, the procedure may be carried out as an emergency, with a view to opening up the artery by angioplasty. The result is similar to that of the clot-busters, which are the far more usual treatment. Alternatively, angiography may be carried out if the woman continues to experience severe pain in the days following a heart attack. This is to assess whether angioplasty or surgery would be appropriate. In many cases, however, the patient stabilizes with standard medication.

Recuperation in Hospital

Following an uncomplicated heart attack, the woman is likely to be sitting out of bed the next day. She should be able to eat and drink normally within 24 hours. The aim will be to encourage her to walk a little further each day, so that she will be fit enough for discharge within about five to seven days. This approach has been found to be of greater benefit than resting in bed.

A treadmill exercise test (*see page 54*) may be performed prior to discharge to assess whether the patient is well enough to go home. Alternatively, it may be carried out a few weeks after discharge to see how well she has recovered. The result would be taken into consideration when deciding whether further investigation by coronary angiography is needed.

Anxieties

Anyone who has had a heart attack will be anxious about the possibility of having another and so may suffer a severe loss of confidence. Such people are inevitably at increased risk, but the chances of surviving for many years can be greatly improved by reducing risk factors and making lifestyle changes. Rehabilitation programmes can help to restore confidence and ensure that the maximum quality of life possible is regained. In the longer term, regular medical checks will help to indentify those who may be at greater risk of having another heart attack.

Heart Failure

Although many people make a good recovery from a heart attack, there is a possibility of a larger one resulting in 'heart failure'. The area of heart muscle which was deprived of blood dies and forms a scar which can reduce the efficiency of the heart's function. When this happens, the circulation of blood (and therefore oxygen) around the body and lungs is impaired, which contributes to the symptoms of heart failure.

The main symptom is shortness of breath, initially on exertion, but if the condition worsens it may eventually come on even at rest. Fluid retention in the tissues leads to swollen ankles. Fatigue is also an early symptom which can worsen. As we said in Chapter 2, it is easy to ignore early symptoms and just put them down to being unfit or growing older, but medication can help. Sometimes symptoms of heart failure occur in hospital following a heart attack or they may develop months or even years later. There may also be angina.

Heart failure can be assessed with echocardiography. The same procedure is used as for stress echocardiography (described in Chapter 4), but without giving any drug that simulates exercise. Echocardiography shows how the heart muscle is contracting, the size of the left ventricle (the chamber which pumps blood to the body) and whether there has been any enlargement of the heart.

A number of drugs are used in the treatment of heart failure which act in different ways to help relieve the symptoms. Diuretics reduce the fluid build-up by making you pass more urine. ACE inhibitors and nitrates help to improve the action of the heart, as does digoxin (a modern version of digitalis, the original remedy derived from foxgloves).

Heart Transplantation

In patients with severe heart failure (which can also have causes other than coronary artery disease), transplantation with another heart may be the only option. Unfortunately, there are far too few organ donors, so there are many criteria used when selecting potential recipients. A patient's age would be taken into consideration, for example, as would any damage to other vital organs. A heart transplant thus remains an operation available to relatively few people.

Health-care professionals, medical charities and governments are endeavouring to educate the public so that the immense value of donating hearts – and other vital organs – is better understood (although the law regarding donation varies in different countries). As leading heart surgeon Professor Sir Magdi Yacoub says, 'Following a successful heart transplant, the benefits in terms of quality of life are amazing. Someone who could scarcely cross a room before the operation would be able to climb stairs two at a time. A new heart can enable the recipient to lead a normal life again.'

Heart transplants are carried out in specialist centres. A woman accepted onto a waiting list would receive comprehensive advice, support and information. 'Patients and their families can contact us whenever they wish before and after the operation. We're very open and try to provide whatever help is needed,' says Andy Cox, Senior Nurse Manager of the Transplant Clinic at world-famous Harefield Hospital. In addition, patients may be able to attend a support group or talk to other people living in their area who have had a transplant.

When a suitable heart becomes available, the actual operation is relatively straightforward and, for the patient, not unlike CABG. A heart-lung bypass machine takes over the work of the heart during transplantation. The diseased heart is removed, leaving enough of the atria (upper heart chambers) to allow the atria of the new donor heart to be stitched to them. The major blood vessels are then reconnected and the new heart can take over from the machine.

Care after the operation differs from routine CABG mainly because the body will try to reject the new heart, and this must be controlled by medication. Our body's natural defence against infections is called the immune system. Its role is to destroy harmful invaders, which it identifies as being 'foreign'. It does not, however, distinguish between these aliens and a donor organ. The result is that a transplanted heart will be attacked in much the same way. Medication that suppresses the immune system (immunosuppressants) therefore has to be taken for life. Virtually everyone who has a heart transplant will experience rejection episodes; these are particularly likely to occur in the six months following the operation. It is therefore necessary for routine hospital tests to be carried out at regular intervals so that if there is evidence of rejection, treatment can be given as early as possible. The patient will also be instructed in how to recognize signs of rejection.

A consequence of taking immunosuppressants is that resistance to infection is reduced. The patient is particularly susceptible in the first three months following transplantation, when drug doses are high. Any infection which occurs can be treated with antibiotics; advice will be given on how best to minimize the risks in the longer-term.

Rehabilitation programmes are of great value to transplant patients, not only in enabling them to derive maximum benefit from the operation, but in encouraging them to lead a healthier life which will help prevent the new heart from becoming diseased.

Advances in Treatment

At the time of writing, very promising advances in the treatment of serious heart failure are being made. An artificial heart, known as a Ventricular Assisted Device (VAD), is being assessed. It is connected to the heart and does most of the pumping work of the left ventricle, powered by batteries worn outside on a belt. It has previously been used to tide some patients over until a donor heart becomes available. Now the hope is that it can remain permanently in place, so that patients retain their own heart.

Another promising development is called cardiomyoplasty. Although not yet widely available, it holds out great hope. The procedure involves using the patient's shoulder muscle (the *latissimus dorsi*) to strengthen the ailing heart. In the first such operations carried out, the muscle was wrapped round the heart and then stimulated with a modified pacemaker to make it behave just like healthy heart muscle. Now a further development is being researched in which an additional heart chamber is created from the same muscle. This works alongside the failing original, boosting blood supply to the body.

Because the patient's own tissue is used, there are no rejection episodes and immunosuppressants are unnecessary. It would also be a more suitable treatment for older men and women for whom a transplant is unsuitable. The first British patient to have cardiomyoplasty was able to resume swimming, gardening and going for walks, whereas before he was virtually immobilized. 'To use your own tissue is a brilliant idea,' he said. 'You feel that you have helped to heal yourself.'

Chapter 6

RECOVERY AND
REHABILITATION

Although recovery from heart surgery or a heart attack begins in hospital, women can face a number of major challenges while recuperating at home. They can be helped, and can help themselves, to meet these challenges so that the best quality of life possible after treatment is attained. Adjusting to a healthier lifestyle is most important of all in maintaining quality of life, and in helping to prevent further problems.

Advice and Support

Advice on recovery at home will be given in hospital and there may be literature, tapes and videos available. It is particularly important for a woman's partner, family or other carers to be involved. The emotional stress on those close to her can be immense, and they will have responsibility for her when she leaves hospital. They need advice and support as much as she does.

The hospital may have a helpline number which can be called whenever necessary. The family doctor is on hand too, not only to continue medical supervision of recovery, but also to give advice and support. There may be a local support group for heart patients and their carers where problems can be shared and encouragement given. Heart charities (*see Useful Addresses*) also offer information and help on how a 'new start' can be made.

About four to six weeks following CABG, angioplasty or a heart attack, patients will have a hospital check-up with the specialist responsible for their treatment (although transplant patients require more frequent checks). This is an opportunity to discuss any problems concerning recovery. Heart specialists can be immensely sympathetic, caring and experienced in dealing with patients' problems. However, other health-care professionals – nurses, dieticians, physiotherapists, social workers and counsellors – are also available to assist in recovery.

An increasing number of hospitals now run cardiac rehabilitation programmes for out-patients, which begin after an initial convalescence period. They are of immense value in speeding recovery, and the benefits are described later in this chapter.

At Home

As a woman recovering at home after heart treatment, what advice would the hospital give you prior to discharge, and what are the challenges you may face?

Whether you have had surgery or angioplasty, the advice regarding dietary changes and quitting smoking would be the same as before treatment. You would again be urged to stop smoking, if you had not already done so. This advice would apply after a heart attack too. Ideally, none of us should smoke and all of us should eat a healthy diet, whether or not we have heart disease. Since the next chapter is written for every woman who wants a healthy heart, we will advise on these matters further there.

Beneficial Exercise

The ultimate aim of recovery is to reach your full physical potential so that you can lead as active a life as possible. We will describe how you should approach activity following surgery or a heart attack, and then look at how women tend to respond to this advice.

Take things quietly for the first few days after returning home and allow others to wait on you. Then do a bit more each day, if you can. Begin by moving around your home at the same level of exercise as when you left hospital. Walking is the best activity in early convalescence as it is gentle and takes you out into the fresh air. It makes sense not to go out in the cold initially, as it can bring on angina in some patients. Start on the flat and walk only a short distance, and go with someone to give you confidence. Increase the distance and build up to a brisk pace during subsequent walks. Even after angioplasty, which can bring about immediate improvements, you may need to build up to being more active.

Certain types of exercise, in addition to brisk walking, are particularly good for recovering heart patients. Swimming is excellent because the whole body is supported by water while being exercised, so there is no stress or jarring. Following surgery, however, women may be concerned about showing their scars. Swimming as part of a rehabilitation programme can help them to come to terms with their appearance.

Cycling is also good, whether on a stationary exercise bike or in the fresh air (but not on congested roads where there is exhaust pollution). It does not stress the upper body and encourages deep breathing.

In each case, exercise should be begun gently and gradually increased, although in older people other physical problems, such as arthritis, may also influence what they can do. Jogging, golf and tennis are more energetic activities which may be possible and are also beneficial. Weight training, and vigorous exercise involving bursts of strenuous activity, should be avoided at this stage because they cause sudden surges in blood pressure.

Heart function in healthy people is improved by increasing the amount of exercise they take (*see Chapter* 7). In those recovering from heart disease, exercise can improve the capacity of a damaged heart. Exercise encourages collaterals to open up; these small blood vessels in the heart can then help to supply the heart muscle with oxygenated blood. The circulation is improved by exercise and the resting heart rate is reduced.

As you increase the amount of exercise you take, you are likely to feel discomfort around your chest, neck, shoulders or back after surgery. This is due simply to the healing process. You may also feel a little breathless, but this should improve with exercise. The same is often true after a heart attack. If breathlessness does not improve it may be due to 'heart failure' (as explained in Chapter 5) and needs medical attention.

Treadmill exercise testing in hospital can help in planning a home exercise programme suited to the individual. However, patients recovering from surgery or a heart attack can particularly benefit from supervised exercise, which is a vital part of a rehabilitation programme.

Housework

Begin light housework when you feel able, though you must not put stress on your arms and shoulders. This means you can do such things as dusting, tidying, cooking, washing dishes and ironing – but you shouldn't vacuum, turn mattresses or carry anything heavy, such as shopping. Follow the hospital's advice about the length of time needed before you can resume such activities. This may be about a couple of months.

You can go shopping, but always use a supermarket trolley/cart, not a handbasket, unless you are buying only a few light items. You will need help loading heavy shopping into the car and unloading it when you get home. Driving is not recommended until after your first hospital check-up, so someone must chauffeur you during this time. If you do not have a car, you could use a trolley bag (a shopping bag on wheels). There are some attractive designs now, so it doesn't have to look geriatric. Many experts consider that everybody should have one for heavy shopping to relieve stress on the back.

When you are fit for heavy lifting again, always do it correctly. Get as close to the object as possible. If it is on the ground, squat down beside it, or go down on one knee, whichever is easier. Lift holding it close to you, using your arm and shoulder muscles, not your back muscles, to avoid back strain. (Exercises to strengthen your arms and shoulders are very important.) Never bend from the waist and haul the object up, and don't lift anything so heavy it really is a struggle.

If you enjoy gardening, confine yourself to pruning and light weeding. Don't do any digging, mowing or hedge-cutting before you're fully recovered. Heavy garden work is notorious for causing back trouble and other problems in perfectly healthy people, so you always need to be careful.

Challenges

There is again far less information on how women actually fare during recovery than on men. However, the limited evidence is that women heart patients are not good at adhering to the kind of advice just given. We have referred to a recent Canadian study of women undergoing heart surgery, and the central part which 'preserving the self' played in helping them to cope. Their sense of self was derived from the ability to fulfil their role in life and from having trusting, supportive relationships.

Not surprisingly, these women felt very fragile on first returning home. They had, as they expressed it, 'lost their glue' (their sense of self) through experiencing physical, mental and emotional turmoil. Recovery involved 'finding the glue' through successfully carrying out daily tasks. They mostly saw their ability to do housework as the measure of their progress. This was often a frustrating and depressing time because they couldn't do much and felt out of control. In one case, the woman 'got sick and tired of being sick', so went against 'doctor's orders' and did things she had been advised against. This may also be a way of denying the seriousness of the health problem and so lessening its impact.

Among the challenges women can face, therefore, is accepting that housework should not be done at the time when they are meant to be taking it easy. There are several reasons why this may be difficult for them. Many women say they feel guilty if they don't do the chores. They often resist help from their family, feeling selfish if they place their health above their caring role. They can also feel vulnerable because others might think they just aren't trying hard enough. This is particularly true of younger women; older women find it easier to accept help from others.

In contrast, men recovering from heart treatment are more able to take things easy and suffer less guilt about it. They are also more likely to go for walks and take other forms of exercise. Women tend to increase their level of activity simply by doing more housework.

Women's behaviour during recovery isn't simply the result of their own inability to accept the situation, however. They do tend to receive less support than men. This may be because a male partner's work prevents him from helping, or he may have difficulty coping with the situation anyway. Although we hear much about 'new men', who are acknowledging the more nurturing 'feminine' side of their nature, not all men can adjust easily to illness in a partner and the role changes it brings.

Family members may expect a woman to resume her domestic role sooner than they would expect a man to go back to work. After heart treatment, men's families tend to wait on them longer, and a frequent complaint is that female carers are overprotective. Research also indicates that many women don't see housework as strenuous – another reason why they may try to begin it before they are really ready.

On the positive side, however, it does seem that women are less likely to become 'cardiac cripples' than men. These are patients who need particular encouragement to resume an active life because they develop a morbid fear of any exertion in case it puts their heart under too much stress.

This research examined the pressures experienced by women in a traditional homemaking role. Fewer women who also work outside the home return to their jobs than men. This may be because of the older age at which heart disease generally occurs in women and/or because they are less likely to be the sole earners. Now, however, the number of women earners whose incomes are essential is increasing, either because they are the family breadwinners or because they are self-supporting. Under normal circumstances, women who work and run the home can feel under pressure to prove they can do both well. They could face even greater challenges during recovery.

Understanding

It is very important for carers to try to understand the impact a heart problem can have on a woman. In a few cases, surgery can bring about personality changes, and research is currently being carried out into why this occurs. Having trusting, supportive relationships with their carers evidently helps women to accept that their physical limitations are normal and must not be a source of stress or guilt. Such support plays a significant part in encouraging their recovery and in motivating them to make lifestyle changes.

In order to 'move on' from the experience of heart treatment, women need to have a sense of gaining control of their lives. The more they are able to preserve their sense of self by these means, the more positive their attitude to treatment and recovery. Without this, women may not benefit fully from successful treatment.

Loving Relationships

It hardly needs saying that heart disease and its treatment will have a profound effect on all aspects of a partnership. However, it is perhaps where sexual relations are concerned that the most confusion, stress and fear exists for women and their partners. There can be the fear that intercourse will bring on pain and even a heart attack. If a woman has had a heart attack, the fear that sex may prove to be fatal is likely to be even greater.

What does research tell us about the sex lives of women who have been treated for heart disease? Predictably, few surveys have been carried out, whereas much more is known about how heart disease and its treatment affect male sexual desire and performance. American studies of women who have had heart attacks show that sexual intercourse is either not resumed or reduced in frequency afterwards. One study of 130 women revealed that 27 percent did not resume their sex life, and in 44 percent it was reduced. Sex can also be less pleasurable. Although both men and women heart patients report being fearful of resuming their sex lives after all forms of treatment, it apparently presents more difficulties for women. Those who restart are slower to do so than men. Because supportive relationships are of such importance in recovery, a partnership in which sexual fulfilment is reduced or absent could impede a woman's progress.

Self-Image and Sexual Problems

In addition to these fears, it may be that surgery has made a woman feel less confident of her attractiveness and femininity. A heart operation leaves a scar running between the breasts – normally an erotic part of a woman's body. Initially, flakes of skin and suture material fall away from it, as a part of healing, but it usually heals to a fine line, which is noticeable though not unsightly. In a full-breasted woman, particularly if she is overweight, the 'pull' on the scar can widen it. Sometimes the scar tissue itself thickens (called keloid scarring) and this is more likely to affect black women. There will also be a scar on the inside of the leg in women who have had CABG.

Women usually change the way they dress to hide the scars, and stylish clothes can have sex appeal without being revealing. Self-image does not seem to be so much of a problem for men. Male clothing and body hair hide scars, which may be part of the reason. Some women, however, may find it easier to accept what has happened to them by not hiding the result.

After a transplant, medication which prevents rejection of the new heart can cause an increase in hair on the face and arms (though not the rest of the body). This can be removed by waxing and depilatory creams, but not by shaving because of the risk of infection via any cuts.

Other female operations which affect a woman's femininity, such as hysterectomy (removal of the womb) and mastectomy (breast removal), can have a profound impact. Women can need time to grieve and come to terms with what has happened to their body. There can be a similar reaction to heart surgery and also to a heart attack, even though it leaves no scars. Feelings of anger and resentment about having heart disease are common, especially if the woman has tried to lead a healthy life ('Why me?'). Scars can be a constant reminder and become a focus for these feelings. Perhaps a partnership has suffered as a result of the pain and fatigue of heart disease. Shared interests may have had to be abandoned, and a woman who feels debilitated may care less about her appearance anyway.

Because heart disease is more likely to develop after the menopause, there may be additional physical difficulties which affect a woman's sex life. Vaginal dryness and urinary problems can occur due to diminished levels of the 'fertility' hormone oestrogen. Taking HRT will help resolve these problems and, as we have said before, may benefit the heart. Other disabilities, which may simply result from ageing, will naturally affect all forms of activity, but do not necessarily prevent sex. It may be a matter of adapting lovemaking positions.

A younger woman with heart disease may worry about suitable contraception, as she should not take the combined pill. The progestogen-only pill and other non-hormonal forms of contraception would be acceptable, however.

Certain medications that may be prescribed to heart patients – such as antihypertensives, antidepressants and sleeping pills – can adversely affect male sexual desire and performance. Their sexual effects on women are virtually unresearched.

Other serious illnesses can cause fear, anger, depression and, consequently, loss of libido (sexual desire). Even so, it appears that lack of desire may not be the most significant reason why women's sex lives suffer. In a smaller study of 14 women, only 3 reported decreased libido a year after a heart attack and none had lost their orgasmic responsiveness.

Information

A major reason given by women heart patients for the adverse effects on their sex lives is simply lack of information, since the limited amount available is mainly designed to help men. Our society still does not really consider sex a legitimate interest for the sick or ageing, and especially not for sick, ageing women. Another

American study showed that conventional prejudices about women's sex lives, based on age and marital status, can be highly inaccurate. They are no indication of who will need information. This study involved interviewing 58 women, aged from 30 to 88, who were being treated in hospital for angina and heart attacks. Contrary to expectation, only 32 percent of the married women were having intercourse prior to hospitalization, compared with 50 percent of single and divorced women. The oldest sexually active woman was 78.

The majority of all ages – whether single, married, separated, divorced or widowed – wanted informative literature and counselling on sex. These requests were not confined to the sexually active either; those currently without partners were interested, as was a woman of 88. But all the women, particularly the older ones, found it difficult to start a discussion about sex. They felt that a health-care professional should do this.

Doctors, nurses and other professional carers are becoming increasingly aware of the need to ask all heart patients if they require advice and, if they are in a relationship, to involve their partners. Again, a rehabilitation programme can provide an opportunity for sympathetic discussion of any fears or problems in a supportive atmosphere.

Guidance

We can give some general guidance and reassurance here on resuming sexual activity. The most usual way of assessing whether sex can be started is the stair-climbing test. This is not as strange as it sounds. It has been established that the cardiovascular effects of stair-climbing are no greater than those of sexual intercourse. To be more precise, when you can climb two flights of stairs totalling 20 steps in 10 seconds without becoming breathless or experiencing pain, you are fit for lovemaking. Even if you can't manage this, you and your partner may still be able to enjoy sex by adjusting your lovemaking style, so that he is the more active – a role men are more inclined to play anyway. After surgery, wait until the chest has fully healed and feels comfortable.

Just as recovering heart patients are advised to build up their level of activity gradually, the same approach applies to sex. There are no rules about 'how often'. It should be started gently in familiar surroundings which help you feel secure, and where you won't be interrupted by phone calls or other people. As the cold may bring on angina, the room should be warm. Avoid lovemaking positions that put pressure on the chest and restrict breathing. Suitable ones include lying on your side facing or with your back to your partner, sitting astride him or with him kneeling in front of you. Spending time on foreplay will increase the heart rate gradually, and it will peak for only a matter of seconds during orgasm.

Some heart patients experience cardiac symptoms at times during lovemaking. These may be alarming to both partners, but extremely rarely indicate a major problem. From a cardiac standpoint, intercourse is usually safe. The same is true of oral sex, caressing and mutual or solo masturbation. Any chest pain can be prevented by taking nitrate medication beforehand. Beta-blockers can also help prevent symptoms in those who take them regularly. However, it is best to have sex when you feel rested and relaxed.

If you need further reassurance, there is a much-quoted research study on the causes of sudden deaths. During the year in which it was carried out, fewer than 0.1 percent were due to a heart attack occurring during lovemaking. Similar research has revealed that around 80 percent of non-fatal coital coronaries happen to people having sex late in the evening, after heavy eating and drinking, and while doing it with someone other than their regular partner. The moral here is clear!

Expert Help

Patients who cannot resume their sex lives may be helped by specialized counselling from a relationship counsellor or sex therapist. Your doctor or the hospital can refer you, if necessary. Some hospitals have psychosexual therapy clinics which offer expert help. There are also some helpful books available (*see Further Reading*).

Relationships most likely to have difficulties are those where problems, such as lack of communication, already existed and were made worse by illness. A partnership that was loving and supportive before heart disease developed is likely to remain so. We certainly would not want to give the impression, however, that sexual activity is always the most important way in which love can be expressed. What matters is that, whatever the nature of the relationship, those involved feel that it is right for them.

Some experts emphasize the importance of the balance between what they describe as our physical 'worker' heart, which keeps us alive, and our 'feeling' heart, which encompasses our mind and emotions. The two interact and our physical heart is thought to work better when our feelings are positive. Negative emotions and experiences put the physical heart under stress. The next chapter explains more about this concept, but it can be said here that a fulfilling partnership contributes greatly to helping our worker heart recover.

Rehabilitation Programmes

The benefits of enrolling on a formal rehabilitation programme, if possible, have already been stressed. Even if your hospital doesn't run one, you may be able to enrol on a residential course at another hospital. Partners or other carers would also be encouraged to attend with you.

Following surgery or a heart attack, a woman would be recommended to join a rehabilitation programme about four weeks later. After CABG, six to eight weeks is the recommended interval, to allow for healing. And three months gives time after a heart transplant for any early episodes of rejection or infection to be dealt with, so that the woman's condition is stabilized.

A non-residential programme would involve attending for one to three days a week for several weeks. A residential one gives more intensive therapy over a shorter time, usually a week or two, which may particularly suit people who need a quick return to active life. Programmes are attended by men and women together, which encourages mutual support. Specialist transplant centres have rehabilitation programmes, but patients who live at a distance can initially attend for rehabilitation at other hospitals. In their case, however, a formal exercise programme continues at home for about 18 months, to give the new heart the best chance.

Benefits

We have already touched on some major benefits of attending for rehabilitation, but it should be emphasized that everyone can gain. Age, for instance, is no barrier to rehabilitation; it says nothing about a person's potential for recovery from heart disease. A younger person can be more seriously affected than someone older (and vice versa). Even when the possibility of physical improvement may be limited, perhaps due to other disabilities in addition to heart disease, the psychological and educational benefits are still very worthwhile.

To give you a better idea of how you will be helped, we'll describe the week-long residential programme at the London Chest Hospital, which was among the earliest to be established in Britain. Its approach is holistic, covering physical, psychological and social rehabilitation.

Each day begins with a walk in the fresh air. There is an hour's exercise in the gym, supervised by physiotherapists and nurses. This starts with 'warm-up' stretching and is followed by a choice of exercises; each is performed for a minute with a minute's rest in between. These include arm and chest strengthening exercises, stationary bicycling, trampolining, floor work and step-ups. Most can be continued at home without special equipment.

There are also water exercise sessions in the pool, which are a gentle way to regain fitness. These can be helpful in another way to women who have had surgery, as mentioned earlier. This is usually the first time they have publicly exposed their scars and it can be reassuring for them to see that they are not alone.

Whatever the form of exercise, individuals are encouraged to do the best they can, not to compete with each other. The more they find they can do, however, the more it builds their confidence. People who have had heart surgery tend to hunch over self-protectively, and exercise improves their posture.

Relaxation is as important as exercise, since stress is a risk factor in heart disease and anxiety can make angina worse. Recognizing personal stresses and learning relaxation techniques is part of the programme. The next chapter describes a variety of approaches to relieving the stresses likely to affect women.

Education is crucial to succesful rehabilitation. There are sessions with a dietician on healthy eating, with a pharmacist on medication and with doctors and nurses on understanding heart disease and the treatments needed. Identifying each person's risk factors, and encouraging the necessary lifestyle changes, is vital. As we have seen, treatments are not cures and rehabilitation is a lifelong commitment. A rehabilitation programme is simply an introduction to a better life.

Group Support

There are group therapy and counselling sessions where patients and their partners can discuss practical problems and share their anxieties. These are opportunities to express emotions about heart disease, such as guilt. This may be the result of having led an unhealthy life which could have precipitated heart disease, or because the patient realizes how illness has made others around her suffer, or – in the case of a transplant – because someone had to die to enable her to live. Other negative emotions – anger, grief and fear – can also be acknowledged and put in perspective.

But positive feelings can also be expressed. Those who are recovering from heart disease have cheated death. This can bring about a major reassessment of their lives which changes their values, priorities and relationships for the better.

Probably the greatest benefit of rehabilitation comes from this sharing and the support group members give each other throughout the programme. This can be particularly important to women who may otherwise be more isolated at home. The benefits of rehabilitation are rapidly obvious. 'By the end of the week people are much more cheerful and confident,' says Carole Flowers, the Clinical Nurse Specialist who runs the cardiac rehabilitation programme at the London Chest Hospital. 'Those who stay in touch say it has helped them tremendously in their new way of life.'

Encouragement

Despite these advantages, however, it appears that fewer women attend rehabilitation programmes than men, and when they do participate, they are more likely to drop out before completion. Family commitments are the most common reason given.

Men who participate are more likely than women to be accompanied by their partner. This may be because men's work prevents them from going with their partner. If, however, partners and other carers encourage women to enrol, and make every effort to attend with them at least some of the time, women would very probably respond more positively. To conclude with Carole Flowers' words, 'It is the beginning of the rest of their lives.'

Chapter 7

HAVING A HEALTHY HEART

All of us should be concerned about having a healthy heart, so this chapter is as much for women interested in preventing heart disease as for those recovering from it. Everyone, in fact, should try to lead the kind of life recommended on rehabilitation programmes. As we have seen, those who attend become more cheerful and confident, which is how our lifestyle should enable us to feel anyway.

A healthy lifestyle involves eating a balanced diet, taking exercise, reducing stress and not smoking. There is no lack of publicity giving us this good advice. It is the basis of a whole lucrative industry. Despite this, more young women are smoking, an increasing number of women are overweight and there is evidence that women generally suffer more from anxiety and tension than men. We'll examine why the message apparently isn't working and try to make some constructive suggestions.

As a positive start, it can be said that a lifestyle which benefits the heart, and every other aspect of our health, is not about giving up the unhealthy things we enjoy and doing things we don't like. That is a negative approach. A healthy lifestyle is about empowering ourselves, taking control of our own life so that it becomes more rewarding.

Don't Smoke

Since the many serious risks of smoking are well known, why are so many young women becoming smokers, and how can women smokers be helped to stop?

Most smokers start young. Few people enjoy cigarettes initially, but nicotine is highly addictive. Those who persist soon find that relieving the craving becomes relaxing and pleasurable, even though it is actually increasing the body's stress reaction (*see Chapter 3*).

Although boys experiment with smoking slightly earlier than girls do, more girls are regular smokers by the age of about 13. This is the pattern throughout much of the developed world, and it would appear that smoking among women is started largely in the mid-teens. Teenage girls are well aware of the longer-term health risks and the social disapproval smoking incurs, but these disadvantages can quite easily be outweighed by the immediate advantages it is seen as having.

Here are some comments from girls who smoke: 'It's sexy and sophisticated.' 'It's a challenge to the boys.' 'If I didn't smoke, I'd eat instead.' 'If your friends smoke, you'll end up wanting to as well.' 'It makes you feel good, gives you something to do with your hands and calms your nerves, so you're more confident with people.' 'When you're working for exams, it's nice to stop for a relaxing cigarette instead of getting more uptight.' 'Smoking is *cool*. You're thumbing your nose at all the disapproval.'

Self-esteem

Recent research carried out in Britain by Dr Anne Charlton of the Cancer Research Campaign at Manchester University sheds light on an underlying reason why girls, rather than boys, might have the greater need to smoke. She and her colleagues analysed questionnaires from 830 children (407 boys and 423 girls). These revealed that the girls' opinions of their appearance, scholastic achievement and overall self-worth fell steadily between the ages of 11 and 15 – just the time when they are liable to become smokers. There was no such decrease among the boys, whose self-esteem generally remained higher.

Not surprisingly, dissatisfaction with their appearance had the greatest impact on the girls' self-esteem. All magazines aimed at this age group – and at women – present an image of feminine beauty which is unrealistic for most of us at any age. The few super-models and other slender celebrities who embody this image are frequently shown smoking. This perpetuates its 'Hollywood glamour' and reinforces the widely held but false belief that it helps in weight loss. These associations are promoted by the advertising industry which presents cigarettes themselves as elegantly slim and smooth as silk.

There are no similar publications or advertisements aimed at teenage boys. They probably do not worry about their appearance to anything like the same extent. It seems they are more likely to smoke if their father or brother does. Family influence on children is strong, and both boys and girls are twice as likely to smoke if their parents do, but about seven times less likely to do so if their parents express disapproval – even when the parents themselves are smokers.

If parents seem not to mind, however, children are more inclined to smoke – even if the parents themselves are non-smokers. A firmer approach is therefore much more effective than a liberal attitude and simply 'setting a good example'. Being firm is actually a way of caring. If children know that their parents are concerned about what they do to themselves, this does help to raise their self-esteem, although girls apparently become more vulnerable to outside influences.

Achievement

Underachievers are more likely to smoke than people who see themselves as successful, but the girls' low opinion of their scholastic achievement was not necessarily a reflection of their real capabilities. The way they saw themselves could have resulted from low self-esteem, or may have been a rejection of the whole idea of achievement – or both.

Many young people rebel against what they see as imposed adult values. Those who 'hate school' are often smokers. Because it is considered unacceptable, smoking can be a way of expressing rebelliousness and building a kind of self-esteem within a group of like-minded friends. (This may be part of the challenge to boys: the girls are daring to smoke when men are giving it up.) As girls themselves say, friends smoking and the desire to be accepted socially are among the most significant factors affecting whether or not they smoke. A girl's family, friends and school all influence self-esteem.

Laying the Foundations

It is at this stage that the foundations can be laid for adult smoking and future health problems, such as heart disease. According to researcher Dr Bobbie Jacobson, not only do women smokers feel less self-confident and more dependent on cigarettes than do men, they also see themselves as being under greater stress and having less control over their lives. This further increases their sense of dependence on smoking.

Women, it seems, are more likely than men to smoke because they think it helps reduce anxious or angry feelings, which they might otherwise be unable to suppress. Stress relief can therefore be more important for many women than concern about weight, although this usually remains a major factor (see the end of this section for the truth on this matter). These are often the strongest reasons against quitting given by women.

The addiction to nicotine means that smoking usually becomes a deeply ingrained habit. Both men and women smokers can feel that relieving the craving has positive effects on many aspects of their lives. Breaking the physical dependence on nicotine is seen by experts as the key to quitting.

Most women smokers wish they could quit. A 30-year-old television presenter sums up the dilemma: 'I started when I was a teenager. It was due to peer pressure. Smoking is a disgusting habit, but I do enjoy it immensely and I'm hopelessly addicted to nicotine. I wish I'd had more sense when I was younger.'

Not Starting

The reasons why women start and continue smoking are varied and complex. As Dr Charlton says, 'Smoking isn't like the cherry on the cake which can be easily removed, it's more like the fruit inside, and you'd have to unravel someone's life to find all the reasons.'

Raising self-esteem in girls does, however, seem to be an essential way of preventing them from starting to smoke. This would involve schools helping them to make the best of their appearance and, above all, encouraging them to accept themselves as they are. This important aspect of growing up is often neglected. Schools should also set realistic goals which enable each girl to achieve her maximum potential, and success in doing this should be praised.

Rebellion can even become constructive. Young rebels often have a strong sense of justice – schoolgirls shown a film about the effects of tobacco production and smoking in developing countries were amazed and appalled. Adult commercial values were seen destroying the health and environment of the less privileged; this made the girls think about their own behaviour.

We live in a society which gives conflicting messages on smoking. It is vital that parents, educators and governments continue to press for measures which will help and protect all young people.

Quitting

What is the best way for women smokers to quit? There is a vast amount of advice and help available to those who want to give it up, and there are some helpful books for women (*see Further Reading*). But it is the desire to quit – the personal commitment to doing so – which is crucial, together with the confidence to believe that you can succeed. Given what we have said about why women may smoke, how can they find the necessary motivation?

If you are thinking of quitting, ask yourself whether you think you will gain more out of giving up than continuing. Having heart or lung disease means there is a simple choice between a better and longer life if you quit, or the opposite if you don't. But if you are not ill, ask yourself what the consequences will be for yourself and others if you become ill. Perhaps you have early signs of ill health, such as a cough and shortness of breath. These will very likely disappear if you quit.

Consider why you started in the first place, and note the times of the day and the situations in which you need a cigarette. In finding ways of overcoming the craving for nicotine, you will also be helping yourself to deal with any stressful feelings you think it is relieving. Because the effects of nicotine are increasing your stress reaction, smoking is giving only a false sense of control. Perhaps you are aware that cigarettes are really controlling you; by quitting you will become an achiever and be more in control of your life.

Methods

There are many approaches to quitting and you need to find which will be best for you, but we can make some suggestions. Generally speaking, simply stopping smoking completely is more likely to be successful than gradually cutting down, where there is the possibility of building up again. It can also be more effective than using products which make cigarettes taste foul.

You can try quitting by yourself or with the support of others who want to give up, which is usually easier. Maybe you have a friend or relative who wants to quit, or you can join a support group; your doctor or hospital may run a group or can put you in touch with one. Heart and cancer charities also offer help and some have telephone 'quitlines' you can call for advice.

Whether you decide to go it alone, or with someone else, try the following steps:

- Choose a 'quit day' when you're not going to be under stress.
- Tell everyone you're giving up so they can encourage you, and ask any smokers not to smoke near you or offer you cigarettes, even on special occasions.
- Throw out your own cigarettes, lighters and ashtrays.

- Change your routine and keep busy to distract yourself from the craving. Acupuncture, hypnotherapy, deep breathing and other relaxation techniques described later may help by relieving stress, as can taking regular exercise.
- Don't say 'I'm quitting forever'. Take it day by day. Each 'smoke free' day is an achievement.
- Save your cigarette money to buy yourself a reward.

Nicotine Replacement Therapy

Some people find quitting surprisingly easy, but for others the sudden loss of nicotine causes severe cravings and unpleasant withdrawal symptoms; these can include irritability, headaches and a sore throat. Using some form of nicotine replacement, such as a skin patch or chewing gum, can help you through the worst effects of quitting.

The patch releases smaller amounts of nicotine into the bloodstream via the skin than would come from cigarettes, and the chewing gum has the same effect. By gradually using smaller patches you are weaned off the need for nicotine. If you already have heart disease, pains in the chest or persistent indigestion, or are taking another medication regularly, you need to consult your doctor before using this therapy. You cannot use it if you are pregnant or breast-feeding.

If you don't manage to quit, you are certainly not alone in finding smoking a tough habit to break. It is always worth another try. A support group can be particularly helpful to those who are trying again.

Worries About Weight

Although it is false, the belief that smoking controls weight is so widely held, especially by women, that some reassurance is needed. The stress reaction to nicotine raises metabolism (the rate at which the body uses energy from food), but the effect on weight is slight.

Some people claim that smoking suppresses their appetite, but this is probably because of its effect on taste. Food may have more flavour after quitting and so ex-smokers may be more inclined to eat, but there is nothing wrong with gaining a small amount of weight if you are not overweight. The average weight gain in quitters is only about 2 kg (4 lb) and this can easily be lost by sensible eating and exercise.

If you're worried that you'll overindulge in fattening 'comfort foods', or you simply need something to put in your mouth, cut some vegetable sticks from carrots or celery and keep them to hand as if they were chocolates or cigarettes.

A final word to the worried: studies carried out in the USA and Holland have shown that some of the women who smoked the most cigarettes also weighed more than either non-smokers or ex-smokers. Weight is controlled by a healthy diet and exercise, as explained next, not by smoking.

Eat and Drink Healthily

A diet low in fat and sugar and high in fibre, and which contains plenty of fresh fruit and vegetables, is widely recommended, together with moderate drinking. This is the healthy way to successful weight control, which will benefit your heart.

As explained in Chapter 3, being very overweight increases the likelihood of developing high blood pressure, high cholesterol and diabetes – all major risk factors for heart disease. If smoking is added, perhaps in the false hope that it will help in weight control, the risk of heart disease becomes very great. In women who already have any of these risk factors, being very overweight will make them even worse. A healthy diet is also vital for those facing heart surgery; being in the best possible shape lessens the trauma and helps speed healing. And it is of immense benefit to those recovering from heart disease.

There is evidence that certain foods can help protect your heart and arteries, and we will be giving information on them, together with guidance on healthy eating. But first we'll look at why the message on diet isn't working.

Missing the Message

The pressures on women to be slim are enormous, and there is a vast amount of dietary advice available, yet the number of over-weight women in developed countries is increasing. (There are more overweight men too, and although they are also advised to reduce, the pressures on them to do so are less.)

There are various possible explanations for this trend. Most convincing is the view, which has rapidly gained ground, that dieting itself is often to blame, together with unhealthy eating habits. Inevitably, the slender, sexy stereotype is again held responsible for millions of women being dissatisfied with their appearance and thinking they need to diet, even when they are not overweight.

Dieting, unfortunately, is not always the same as eating health-ily. The energy the body uses, and the amount of food needed to provide it, is measured in calories. As already mentioned, the metabolic rate is the speed at which the body uses energy from food by 'burning up' calories. Low-calorie diets involve cutting down drastically on foods over a short period of time and/or using meal replacements, usually in the form of snack bars, soups and milkshakes.

Rapid weight loss can be achieved as the body 'burns' stored fat as energy, but in the vast majority of women the weight is then regained because the diet does not change the unhealthy eating habits, which are resumed. Worse still, because many diets involve completely giving up certain favourite foods (such as chocolates and cream cakes), there is then the temptation to binge on them when they are 'allowed' again.

Going on another diet then becomes necessary, and a vicious circle of dieting and regaining often sets in. This is referred to as 'yo-yo dieting' or 'weight recycling'. It is physically and psycholog-ically dangerous.

Dangers

With repeated dieting, the metabolic rate slows and adjusts to using fewer calories. When dieting is discontinued, more weight is regained each time because less food is needed by the body for energy. In addition, muscle tissue as well as fat can be lost. It is important to maintain muscles through exercise because they burn up energy in use, and exercise is also good for the heart in ways we shall describe later in this chapter.

Other drastic weight-loss methods are often similarly ineffective in the longer term. These include diet pills, jaw-wiring (which permits only a liquid diet) and surgical ways of removing fat. They do not change eating habits or involve healthy exercise.

Many overweight women are failed dieters, either because they could not stick to dieting or because they regained weight anyway afterwards. This can make them feel depressed, guilty and inadequate; it may cause an obsession with foods which supposedly can or cannot be eaten; and it disrupts the pleasures of cooking, eating and sharing a meal with others.

It is this kind of failure and misery, coupled with the social rejection of fat people, which has caused some larger women to abandon the whole business of dieting and to campaign for 'fat acceptance'. They wish their size to be seen as normal for them.

While it is never right to hurt and embarrass people because of their size, being very overweight is associated not only with heart disease, but also with other health problems. These include arthritis, gallstones, strokes and some female cancers, such as cancer of the breast and womb. This isn't to say that if you are large you will inevitably become ill but, whatever our size, we all need to be aware of factors which could affect our health.

Other Culprits

Dieting cannot be blamed entirely for the increase in the number of overweight people, however. Diseases which cause obesity are rare, and there are numerous other reasons why women may put on weight.

Decreased physical activity and the increased availability of tempting high-energy foods, rich in fat and sugar, are probably the most important factors. Unhealthy eating may be a response to psychological and emotional stresses. A feminist view is that being overweight can be a protest against the inequality of the sexes – a rejection of the slender, sexy stereotype which appeals to men. An eloquent advocate of fat acceptance touches on some complex aspects: 'I eat when under pressure; I eat when I am upset or worried ... I believe that every woman's reason for being fat, whether she understands it or not, is her own, related to her own personality and personal circumstances.'*

Slimness

Some of us, on the other hand, put on weight more easily than others, and genetics (inherited characteristics) play a part in our shape and size. Supermodel slimness is certainly not healthy or realistic for the majority of women. Some women are naturally slim and healthy, but being more rounded can be healthy too.

The proportion of fat is what matters. Between 18 and 30 per cent of weight in a healthy woman should be fat. Female fat has some important functions. The 'fertility' hormone oestrogen is produced by the ovaries and independently in body fat. As we have said in previous chapters, it is thought to help protect women from heart disease prior to the menopause. Very thin women are more likely to have an early menopause, particularly if they smoke.

Infertility can result at an early age if too much body fat is lost, and the heart can be affected. Extreme dieting, as occurs in anorexia nervosa (self-starvation), can cause periods to stop due to the lack of oestrogen. This eating disorder affects mainly girls and young women. If anorexia is not treated successfully, it is sometimes fatal.

Bulimia nervosa (bingeing followed by self-induced vomiting), is often a variant of anorexia. It can cause abnormalities in the heartbeat due to the loss of the mineral potassium, which helps to maintain normal heart rhythm. Like anorexia, it also has other extremely serious consequences.

Anorexia and bulimia have complex underlying psychological causes. Young women affected often see dieting as a way of con-

* In *The Forbidden Body*, Shelley Bovey (Pandora, 1994)

trolling their lives. The fear of weight-gain is a major factor and these disorders are on the increase. Professional help is almost always needed to treat them.

Acceptable Weights

Maintaining a stable weight is the best way to stay healthy, and there is an acceptable weight range for your height. The following chart gives the British Heart Foundation recommendations (add 2 kg/4 lb if you weigh yourself in clothes).

Height		Acceptable Weight Range	
1.25 m	(4 ft 11 in)	42.6–55.3 kg	(94–122 lb)
1.52 m	(5 ft 0 in)	43.5–56.7 kg	(96–125 lb)
1.55 m	(5 ft 1 in)	44.9–58 kg	(99–128 lb)
1.57 m	(5 ft 2 in)	46.2–59.4 kg	(102–131 lb)
1.60 m	(5 ft 3 in)	47.6–60.7 kg	(105–134 lb)
1.63 m	(5 ft 4 in)	48.9–62.5 kg	(108–138 lb)
1.65 m	(5 ft 5 in)	50.3–64.4 kg	(111–142 lb)
1.68 m	(5 ft 6 in)	51.7–66.2 kg	(114–146 lb)
1.70 m	(5 ft 7 in)	53.5–68 kg	(118–150 lb)
1.73 m	(5 ft 8 in)	55.3–69.8 kg	(122–154 lb)
1.75 m	(5 ft 9 in)	57.1–71.6 kg	(126–158 lb)
1.78 m	(5 ft 10 in)	58.9–73.9 kg	(130–163 lb)
1.80 m	(5 ft 11 in)	60.7–76.2 kg	(134–168 lb)
1.83 m	(6 ft 0 in)	62.5–78.4 kg	(138–173 lb)

In Chapter 3 we explained how to calculate your BMI (body mass index) by dividing your weight in kilos by your height in metres squared (*see page 41*). A BMI of over 30 is obese and the likelihood of developing risk factors for heart disease is then much greater. As we also indicated, the distribution of fat matters too. Women who carry most of their excess weight around their middle – as often happens after the menopause – run a higher risk of heart disease. Your waist/hip ratio is therefore important. To calculate this, measure your waist and hips, then divide the waist measurement by the hip measurement. The answer should be under 0.8 or you are at increased risk.

If you are obese, you should take advice from your doctor or a nutritionist s/he recommends. Some hospitals run weight reduction clinics and there are also commercial organizations offering programmes, but you should only attend those which are reputable and approved by your doctor or hospital. Medical supervision is needed for any diet under 1,000 calories a day. Anyone who needs to lose weight should do so gradually. Avoid diets that promise weight loss of more than 1 kg (2 lb) per week and those that do not offer healthy nutritional advice.

Calories

Excess calories obtained from food are stored as fat, so eating an appropriate number of calories controls weight. It is estimated that women generally need 1,700–2,400 calories per day, depending on how active they are. The information given on food labels is improving, and the calorie content is usually expressed as the number per 100 g (the number of calories per serving may also be given).

Calories are often called kilocalories (kcal); kilojoules (kJ) are the metric equivalent and there are about four to each kilocalorie. Foods that contain fewer than 100 kcal per 100 g are low-calorie; those with more than 250 kcal per 100 g are high-calorie. While it is helpful to be aware of the calorie content of different foods, it is not necessary to count calories slavishly to control weight if you eat healthily.

Healthy Eating

It is much more beneficial to take a holistic approach to eating and weight control so that they are a part of a healthy lifestyle, rather than a separate preoccupation. Don't treat anything as forbidden, but visualize your diet as forming a pyramid, with foods you should eat least near the top (where we shall start) and those you can have most of at the base.

Sugary Foods

Cakes, cookies, confectionery and pastries are least to be recommended. These high-calorie foods contain refined sugar and are often described as providing 'empty energy' because they have little nutritional value and cause rapid weight gain. They are usually high in fat too, which is often saturated (animal) and so has an adverse effect on lipids. Other foods with added refined sugar, such as canned fruit, also have a much higher sugar content than the levels of natural sugar found in fresh fruit.

Although it is obviously advisable to avoid these foods, you can still eat them occasionally in moderation if you have the urge. Regarding them as 'forbidden' is often what leads to bingeing. Popular and widely available, they form part of social celebrations – and our quality of life matters too.

Fats and Oils

All fats and oils are high-calorie energy-givers containing, on average, 9 calories per gram. As many of us are aware, the distinction between saturated fats of animal origin and unsaturated (non-animal) fats is important for the heart and arteries. Saturated fats are usually hard at room temperature. Lard (cooking fat), butter (and also whole milk and cream), full-fat cheeses and red meat are high in them and they are implicated in raising lipid levels, particularly in women after the menopause.

Unsaturated fats are liquid vegetable oils (except for coconut and palm oil, which are saturated). There are two types of unsaturated fats: polyunsaturated and monounsaturated, both of which have a beneficial effect on lipids. Polyunsaturated fats lower the general level of cholesterol and are found in sunflower, safflower, soya, grapeseed and walnut oil. Monounsaturated fats, however, seem to be more discerning in that they lower 'bad' LDL cholesterol levels while promoting higher levels of 'good' HDL cholesterol (*see page 37*). Almond, avocado, peanut, ground-nut, rapeseed and olive oil are rich sources. Corn oil contains about equal proportions of both fats. All these oils are also good sources of the antioxidant vitamin E, which helps 'mop up' free radicals that are thought to promote arterial damage (*see Chapter 3*).

We have been encouraged to use polyunsaturated spreads on our bread rather than butter, but this is now being questioned. The hardening process, called hydrogenation, creates transfatty acids; an American study of 85,000 nurses suggests that a high intake of these may be associated with an increased risk of heart disease, though this has yet to be proved conclusively. An alternative, which is becoming popular, is to use a little olive oil instead of spread.

Dairy products, however, contain the antioxidant vitamin A and are a rich source of calcium, which is necessary for healthy bones and to reduce the future risk of osteoporosis (thinning of the bones) in women after the menopause. They are also a source of protein (described next). Substitutes which meet these needs and have less effect on lipids include low-fat cheeses, yoghurt and fromage frais and skimmed or semi-skimmed milk.

The overall advice here is to use unsaturated oil in cooking and all fats and oils sparingly. They should make up about five percent of your daily diet, bearing in mind that other foods also contain them. But don't entirely deny yourself butter or French cheeses if you like them; enjoy them in small amounts every now and then.

Protein

We need protein for the repair and renewal of cells, and it should form about 20 percent of our diet. Lean meat, fish, milk, cheese and eggs are rich animal souces. Vegetable proteins come from beans, peas, lentils, nuts and cereals, and are found in lesser amounts in most vegetables.

How does protein help your heart? To start with, protein is lower in calories than fat (it contains about 4 calories per gram), although this depends on the form in which it is eaten. Red meat contains more saturated fat than white meat, such as poultry and veal, so if you are not a vegetarian, cut down on red meat and remove the visible fat and the skin from poultry (the fat is under the skin). Meat contains vitamin E, but meat products (sausages, hamburgers, meat pies, pâté) are high in saturated fats and should not form part of your regular diet. Egg yolks are high in fat, but are not as harmful to the arteries as was once thought; they are also a source of vitamins A and E.

Nuts and oily fish contain fat, but this has advantages. The fat is unsaturated, and fish oil is rich in omega-3 fatty acids which lower cholesterol, thin the blood and so help protect against heart disease (the reason why it is rare among Eskimos who eat abundant oily fish). We have described the benefits of nut oils. Because nuts are a rich source of protein and vitamin E, they can replace meat. Include some unsalted nuts and oily fish, such as herring, salmon, mackerel, sardines, tuna, anchovies and whitebait in your diet each week.

Your daily diet should contain fewer than 70 grams of fat from protein and other sources (less then 30 percent of your daily calorie intake), and as much as possible should be unsaturated. Get into the habit of checking food labels so you are aware of the 'hidden fat' in foods.

Carbohydrates

We have reached the base of the pyramid where the bulk of your diet should be made up of unrefined carbohydrates (starches and sugars). These do not include refined sugar and white flour used in the sugary foods described earlier. Vegetables, fruit, wholegrain bread and flours, cereals, rice and pasta all contain unrefined carbohydrates.

Carbohydrates generally have fewer calories than protein and fats (about 3.74 per gram), but are more satisfying for two reasons: the high fibre content adds bulk without increasing calories, so you feel fuller; and they are digested more rapidly, which satisfies the appetite. By contrast, fatty foods don't fill us and take several hours to digest, so we are inclined to eat more of them.

A diet high in unrefined carbohydrates is therefore helpful in reducing both fat intake and weight. It is also of benefit to the heart in other ways because it is a good source of the antioxidant vitamins A, C and E. Carrots, green vegetables, apricots, peaches and plums, for example, contain vitamin A. Citrus fruits, strawberries, kiwi fruit, green peppers, tomatoes, potatoes and leafy vegetables contain vitamin C, which is also thought to help in healing and so may be good for those who have had surgery. Vitamin E is to be found in cereals, wholemeal bread and green vegetables.

(Folic acid, one of the B vitamins, is also obtained from green leafy vegetables, and is increasingly considered to be protective against heart attacks and strokes.) A balanced diet should provide enough of all these nutrients. There is controversy over whether vitamin supplements are helpful (although too much vitamin A can be harmful). Take the advice of your doctor or hospital.

Eating apples every day may reduce the risk of heart disease. They contain antioxidants called flavonoids, also found in red wine (as explained later). So it seems that an apple a day could keep the doctor away! Flavonoids are also found in onions, although the effects are thought to be less.

In addition, the reputation of garlic as a heart-protector is rising. Studies have shown that, when combined with a low-fat diet, garlic supplements may reduce LDL cholesterol and blood pressure. (When taken as powder or capsules they do not make the breath smell.) Garlic's anticoagulant properties are thought to be similar to those of aspirin, so patients on anticoagulants should check with their doctor before taking supplements. The recommended dose should never be exceeded. But do use garlic, herbs and spices as seasonings, rather than salt, which raises blood pressure. Buy food products which are low in salt (sodium) or salt-free, and don't add salt to food on the plate.

The Mediterranean Diet

Our nutritional advice is similar to the popular 'Mediterranean diet', which includes plenty of fresh fruit and vegetables, garlic and olive oil. This diet is of increasing medical interest because it appears to help prevent both cancer and heart disease.

The World Health Organization is studying the connection between diet and heart disease, and has found that the rates in France are far lower than in most industrialized nations. Women in Glasgow, for instance, die of heart disease 12 times more often than those in southern France. Scotland, Finland, northern Europe, the USA and Australia all have much higher rates of heart disease, and their diets are high in fat. Yet the French are not vegetarians, so their lower rates of heart disease have been termed 'the French paradox'. But they do eat far more fresh fruit and vegetables – and they drink wine with meals, which brings us to another important aspect of a healthy diet.

Healthy Drinking

As advised earlier in the book, moderate drinking for women means a couple of small glasses of alcohol a day, but not on an empty stomach. Alcohol is high in calories (there are around 7 per gram), so this is one good reason to drink moderately. Another is the benefit to the heart and arteries. Research has shown that men who drink moderately tend to live longer than either heavy drinkers or non-drinkers, and this is also thought to apply to women.

It seems that all forms of alcohol in modest amounts raise 'good' HDL and lower 'bad' LDL cholesterol. But red wine, which is drunk more often in France than white, also contains the flavonoids mentioned earlier, which are highly protective against the effects of LDL cholesterol. For those who don't like its taste, there are now red wine capsules available to be taken with meals. Some experts also recommend a little dry champagne – not only because it raises our spirits, but because it contains mineral salts which may help protect the heart and arteries. Indian and Chinese 'green tea' (drunk without milk) also contain flavonoids. Green tea is a traditional cholesterol-lowering agent in Chinese medicine.

Feeding the Family

Maintaining healthy eating and a stable weight is a continuous commitment. Understanding how food can give you energy and help your heart puts you more in control. Women, however, often have to satisfy the tastes of a partner and family, and it is not always easy to reconcile healthy eating advice with this.

Providing meals defines women as caregivers and it is important to us emotionally and practically that our food is enjoyed. We suggest that if your family's habits don't include healthy eating, you do not try to change their diet overnight, but simply introduce healthier alternatives. These include the low-fat dairy produce mentioned earlier, more fruit and vegetables, unsweetened fruit juices and diet cola drinks instead of high-calorie, artificially sweetened alternatives. Avoid frying food, bake with wholemeal flour and encourage everyone to eat fresh or dried fruit and nuts as snacks, rather than chocolate bars. When you eat in restaurants, avoid dishes with creamy sauces and, if necessary, ask about ingredients. There is increasing pressure for the nutritional content of food to be given in menus.

Although this book is for women, we so often have responsibility for the health of those close to us. In concluding this section, it is worth mentioning the growing medical concern that junk food, and an inactive 'couch potato' lifestyle, are putting even children aged under 10 at risk of heart disease. To benefit our hearts, we all need not only to eat healthily, but to balance our calorie intake with adequate exercise.

Take Exercise

The type of exercise that benefits the heart is aerobic. It is vigorous enough to make you pant, which stimulates the circulation and strengthens the heart. In the previous chapter we covered the kinds of aerobic exercise to be taken, if possible, during recovery and rehabilitation. These include brisk walking, jogging, swimming, cycling and sports such as golf and tennis. Aerobic exercise is, in fact, heart-improving for everyone in several important ways.

Advantages

We have indicated how exercise helps in weight control through burning calories (energy), and by strengthening muscles which perform this valuable task. As we grow older, we tend to become less active and our metabolic rate decreases. Women are most likely to put on weight in their 50s and 60s, when they also become more vulnerable to heart disease. A major benefit of regular exercise is that it boosts the metabolic rate, so the body continues to use up more calories for a while afterwards.

Chapter 1 explains how taking exercise (or experiencing emotional stress) results in the release of the 'fight or flight' hormones, adrenaline and noradrenaline. They increase the speed and strength of the heartbeat, which raises blood pressure; the breathing rate increases to meet the body's greater demand for oxygen; and stored nutrients – fats and sugars (glucose) – are released into the bloodstream to provide the necessary fuel. Regular aerobic exercise not only burns these up, it also raises the levels of protective HDL, so there is less chance of fats being deposited in the arteries and of clots forming. Research has shown, for example, that a brisk walk before a meal helps reduce fats in the blood afterwards.

In those with heart disease, exercise combined with a lipid-lowering diet can bring about a regression in the atheroma furring up their coronary arteries. Studies of patients with angina have shown that regular, carefully graded exercise taken over a period of time can much improve the pain in some patients and may relieve it entirely in others.

When the 'flight or fight' response is caused by emotional and psychological stresses, regular exercise helps relieve the physical effects by allowing us to 'let off steam'. It reduces high blood pressure, which is particularly associated with heart disease in women, and so is an excellent way to unwind.

Taken regularly, aerobic exercise can directly improve the function of the heart. Like any other muscle, the heart responds to exercise by becoming more efficient, and it may enlarge slightly in a healthy way. This means it can pump more blood with fewer beats and so the resting rate is lower.

If you are very unfit and overweight, have back trouble, joint problems or other disabilities, or risk factors associated with cardiovascular disease (such as high blood pressure, diabetes or circulatory problems), you must discuss with your doctor the type of exercise suitable for you.

Fitness

Taking your own pulse rate is a way of determining how fit you are. Bear in mind that in addition to stress, such things as alcohol, strong tea or coffee and certain drugs can alter the resting rate, so check the effects of any medication you are on and take your pulse in the morning before eating and drinking. This is done by pressing your fingers gently over an artery in either the wrist or the side of the neck and counting the number of beats per minute.

A fit person will have a rate of between 60 and 70 beats per minute; someone less fit will have a rate of 80–90 or even higher. The maximum heart rate you should reach during exercise is calculated by subtracting your age from 220. If you are unfit, don't go above 75 percent of this figure. Take it again about five minutes after you have stopped exercising; it shouldn't exceed 120.

How to Start

If you are not in the habit of exercising regularly, it is best to begin gently (as in cardiac rehabilitation) and gradually build up your fitness. Exercise should be vigorous enough to make you pant, but you should not become so breathless that you are unable to speak. If you feel any pain or get very tired, take it more slowly next time.

Although more women are exercising on a regular basis, many of us still feel that we don't really have the time. Like healthy eating or quitting smoking, exercise does involve making a commitment, but this can simply mean building more activity into your daily life. Start by walking or cycling short distances instead of taking the car. Use the stairs instead of elevators or escalators. It really will make a difference.

Exercise should be enjoyable, a break from routine. There is no lack of books, magazines, tapes and videos to give you ideas about exercise you might enjoy, but ensure that the advice is given by an experienced teacher and suits your level of fitness. Heart charities (*see Useful Addresses*) have their own helpful publications and will recommend other sources of information.

You can do simple exercises at home, with or without exercise equipment. Jogging or running on the spot, for example, can be managed by most of us. Skipping requires only a rope. You could pedal an exercise bike or use a rowing maching while watching television.

Exercise can be an opportunity for an outing with family or friends; exercising with others can help to keep you motivated and be an opportunity to meet new people. Find out what facilities there are locally for swimming, aerobic exercise classes, dancing, sport or gym training (though weight training and sports involving sudden burst of activity – called anaerobic exercise – are not recommended for the heart).

To be effective, aerobic exercise needs to be sustained for about five minutes, and you should aim to have at least three sessions a week, each lasting about half an hour. But if you are exercising with others, don't push yourself to compete with fitter people.

An increasing number of health clubs offer a holistic approach to fitness which combines exercises with advice on relaxation, coping with stress, healthy eating and weight control. They may also offer massage, aromatherapy, yoga and other 'complementary' therapies. Some of these clubs are for women only. Good clubs will assess you on joining, then provide a programme tailored to your needs and given by qualified staff. To get you started, and to help you to stay in shape, you could go to a health farm, if you can afford it. Health farms offer exercise programmes, 'whole body' beauty and relaxation therapies, and usually a vegetarian diet.

Longer-Term Health

Regular exercise builds confidence and gives a sense of achievement. You will look and feel better for it, because what is good for your heart is good for every aspect of your longer-term health and wellbeing.

Reduce Stress

Defining precisely what is meant by stress isn't easy. The word carries negative connotations suggestive of distress, anxiety, frustration and hardship, but not all stress is bad. Many of us relish the excitement of a challenge and a certain amount of stress can bring out the best in us, enabling us to achieve more in life. What is clear is that when the pressures and demands of life become 'too much', our health may be at risk.

Doctors are increasingly taking stress into account when diagnosing and treating problems such as heart disease. But there is much that we ourselves can do to help relieve stresses which may be undermining our health or impeding recovery.

Before we look at ways of reducing stress, it is worth giving further consideration to the kinds of stresses which could be associated with heart disease in women. We touched on them earlier in the book (*see Chapter 3*), but such information as exists is very limited, and further research is urgently needed. Women's role is changing rapidly and with it the stresses it brings. In addition, our perception of what is stressful and our reaction to it will be different for each one of us. It will be influenced by such factors as our genetic makeup and personality, early experiences and present lifestyle. Bearing all this in mind, we should try to be aware of possible stressors in our own lives which could affect our health.

Work and Home

A recent review of the Framingham Heart Study covering 20 years gives some insight into the psychosocial stressors which may be associated with increased risk of heart disease in women. The study surveyed 749 women aged between 45 and 64. Over half had worked outside the home most of their adult lives and the vast majority were married. They were all healthy at the start of the study, but subsequently 69 had heart attacks and there were 10 deaths.

Among employed women, it emerged that those who perceived

themselves to be worse off financially than others were at highest risk of heart attacks. However, another study carried out among healthy young women workers at Cornell Medical Centre, New York Hospital, all of whom had normal blood pressure, showed that the blood pressure became highest during the course of the day in those who found the job itself stressful. Higher pressures also occurred in the women with children (the more children the greater the pressure) due to stress at home. Being overweight and having a family history of hypertension were also factors in the women whose blood pressure rose. Research from Germany has shown that working women with children are far more likely to reach for cigarettes or alcohol in stressful moments than homemakers. Thus a low income and the stress of combining work with homemaking responsibilities may all contribute to the risk of heart disease.

Homemakers, however, can be at risk for other reasons. In the Framingham Study, they had twice the risk of a heart attack if they were lonely during the day, bored, dissastisfied with life, had a poor appetite, difficulty sleeping and disliked housework to the extent that it upset their health. Another study of Alameda County residents in California found that women who lacked social ties had over three times the risk of dying of heart disease compared to women who had many social contacts. This may be a reason why Framingham women who rarely attended religious services were more vulnerable to heart disease. Social support is good for one's health.

Unsurprisingly, homemakers who went without a holiday break for more than six years had double the risk of those who took two or more vacations a year. And those who thought they were likely to develop heart disease were twice as likely actually to do so.

Loneliness, lack of the opportunity or desire to get away and relax, and feeling vulnerable to heart disease were, in fact, associated with heart attacks in all women, but especially in homemakers.

Tension and Anxiety

Compared to the men in the Framingham study, the women experienced greater tension and anxiety, and repressed their angry feelings more. This was particularly true of those employed outside the home, who also apparently had more marital dissatisfaction and worries about ageing. They also had less education, changed their jobs more often and received fewer promotions than the men.

Feeling trapped in unsatisfactory relationships or routine and being under constant pressure from our environment or lifestyle could lead to exhaustion and depression. Studies in men show that depression and fatigue, especially 'waking up exhausted', often precede a heart attack. These symptoms may be the result both of existing heart disease and way of life.

Heart attacks, strokes and sudden death are not usually random events; they tend to occur in the mornings, Monday being the most usual day. Having to return to stressful work is possibly an important trigger in both men and women.

Women in situations where they feel subordinated and isolated are likely to be more prone to heart disease. Nevertheless, personality may also play an important part.

Personality

We hear much about 'Type A and B' personalities in connection with heart disease in men. 'Type A' are described as ambitious, competitive, aggressive, dominating and hard-driving. 'Type B', in contrast, are more relaxed and easy-going. These definitions are now being applied to women.

It comes as no surprise that more Type A women are to be found in the workplace than in the home, and to have white collar managerial jobs. They may, however, be inclined to suppress their Type A characteristics, perhaps because women are traditionally socialized not to behave in a Type A way. This may mean that they are more likely to feel frustrated, irritated and depressed than men. It would appear that Type A people of both sexes are prone to worry, and it was once thought that they were more vulnerable to heart attacks than Type B.

Contrary to this view, research has failed to show a consistent relationship between Type A personality and heart attacks. In the Framingham study, both Types, whether male or female, appear similarly vulnerable, but Type A people of either sex suffer more from chest pain. Whether this is due mainly to angina (pain from the heart) or other causes needs further research. However, Type A people have fewer 'silent' or unrecognized heart attacks (*see Chapter 2*), which may mean that they are more alert to symptoms than Type B.

Naturally, not everyone will fit neatly into the Type A or B pattern. It is therefore very worthwhile taking time out to relax (for a few minutes a day, at the very least). This is especially important if you recognize Type A characteristics in yourself, because Type A people tend to drive themselves too hard.

Emotions and Life Events

In addition to daily stresses, there can be the impact of major life events. Since we are all human beings, these probably have as profound an effect on women as on men. We are familiar with the concept of heartache and even 'dying of a broken heart'. The social readjustment rating scale is a well-known method of evaluating the impact of such events (s*ee Further Reading for books on stress which discuss this in detail*). It places stressors such as bereavement, divorce, loss of job, change in work or retirement high on the list of experiences which could seriously affect health. Some counsellors consider that hurtful past experiences, which may be buried deep within us, could eventually contribute to heartbreak and ill health.

Moreover, early in life we may have been obliged to repress important qualities in ourselves – such as being sensitive, playful or imaginative – so that we are better able to survive in a tough world. This can mean that we do not live fully as our true selves, and this too could undermine us. Early experiences influence the development of our personality. A health crisis, such as heart disease or a heart attack, can lead us to question ourselves deeply, although we should take steps to lead a healthy life before this point is reached.

Gaining insight into our true selves, and finding ways of relieving the stresses which may be affecting us, could be the keys to maintaining a healthy balance between our 'feeling' heart (which encompasses our mind and emotions) and our physical 'worker' heart which keeps us alive. This concept was created by psychotherapist Elizabeth Wilde McCormick and is used in her counselling work with heart patients. It is a poetic way of saying that relaxation and a positive outlook help to balance the sympathetic and parasympathetic nervous systems, described in Chapter 1.

Positive Action

How, then, can a woman help her feeling heart to assist her worker heart? Since women tend to repress negative emotions, which in itself can make stressful situations more stressful, learning to be more positive and assertive could make self-expression and goal-achievement easier. This means being able to handle difficult situations or perceived put-downs in a firm but non-aggressive way, and knowing how to make the most of opportunities.

Employers are more aware that in helping women to develop their managerial skills they will be improving the quality of their workforce. It is therefore well worth attending a staff or management training course if possible. If your employer does not provide these, or you are a homemaker and feel that your self-esteem and confidence need raising, there are assertiveness workshops you can attend. Ask about them at your local adult education college or library. There are also books and tapes on the subject (*see Further Reading*).

We have covered the benefits of exercise in helping you to relax and build confidence. You may find that learning one of the martial arts, such as judo or karate, is not only good exercise but will give you a greater sense of power. Knowing that you can defend yourself if attacked physically could enable you to feel generally less vulnerable in a dangerous world.

Relaxation Techniques

Learning to relax is an important part of becoming more confident and assertive. You will cope better with stressful situations and emotions if you are calm. If you are trying to quit smoking, for instance, relaxation techniques will help you cope with the stresses that make you reach for a cigarette, as well as with the craving for nicotine. If you have angina, or have had a heart attack, they can be valuable both in relieving pain and in preventing its onset.

Simply breathing deeply, if done correctly, is an excellent relaxation technique which can be carried out anywhere in any stressful situation. It brings virtually instant relief by slowing your heart rate and lowering blood pressure, so reducing your natural stress reaction (the 'fight or flight' response). It can, for example, be helpful if you feel anxious prior to any medical procedure.

Here's how to do it. Keeping your back straight, breathe in deeply, filling the lungs using your diaphragm (the muscle between your chest and abdominal cavity). Breathe out slowly, emptying the lungs. Continue to breathe deeply, slowly and regularly. This is how you should always breathe. It prevents the shallow, rapid 'upper chest' breathing called hyperventilation, which results from stress.

This can be combined with the 'Stop' technique. If you feel yourself getting worked up, say 'stop' sharply to yourself, aloud if the situation permits. Then breathe in deeply and out slowly, relaxing your hands and shoulders at the same time. With the next breath, relax your shoulders and jaw. If you have to talk, speak a bit more slowly, with your voice a little lower.

Complementary Therapies

The following information and advice are given by Felicity Smart and John Gold, Complementary Therapist and Counsellor

Correct breathing control is central to yoga and other complementary therapies which will help you relax. These therapies create inner calmness, and some involve counselling to help you recognize stressors and improve your lifestyle.

The most important role of complementary therapies is in

restoring mind, body and spirit to 'wholeness'. This is why they are also called holistic or 'whole-person' therapies. Physical disorders are seen as resulting from a number of factors, such as stress and an unsatisfactory lifestyle. The person is thus in a state of inner disharmony or 'dis-ease'. This interpretation is compatible with orthodox medical views. There are doctors and specialists who remain sceptical about combining these therapies with orthodox approaches. Others consider them a helpful complement, and so they are now less often described as 'alternative therapies'. Complementary therapies aim to help you activate your own inner healing power which, it is believed, we all possess.

Those described here are popular and easily available; they are considered safe, and the heart may benefit through the help they give to the health of the 'whole person'. Some doctors, nurses and other health-care professionals have also trained in complementary therapies, and so can help you themselves. Health clubs may offer them as part of a holistic approach to fitness.

There is a wide range of complementary therapies (*see References and Further Reading for sources of more information*). If you are seeking help independently, contact the organizations that represent the therapies you wish to try (*see Useful Addresses*). They will put you in touch with the nearest fully trained and reputable therapist who, as a member of an organization, will be bound by its code of practice.

It is vital to have a good personal rapport with a therapist. Complementary therapists should not advise you against having orthodox treatment, nor can they offer cures. But there is a strong emphasis on self-help, which means that they place you more in control of your life.

Yoga and Meditation

Some of the best-known therapies originated in the East, where they are part of a philosophy of life. Yoga is one of these. This ancient Indian philosophy combines breathing exercises (pranayama) and postures (asanas) as a preparation for meditation. Yoga is Sanskrit for 'union', which sums up its purpose: to create harmony between mind, body and spirit.

The breathing exercises calm and relax both mind and body, the postures improve flexibility and muscular control, and meditation completes the therapeutic effect. The aim of meditation is to clear the mind of everyday cares, as well as of any deeper anxieties, in order to bring complete inner calm.

To aid meditation, you can focus your mind on a colour, a sound or a positive thought. Hindu meditation, for instance, concentrates the mind on sacred words (called mantras). Couéism is a Western form of meditation named after Emile Coué, the 19th-century French apothecary. The positive power of suggestion is obvious in his famous phrase, 'Every day, in every way, I am getting better and better.' Repeating these words during recovery from heart disease, and allowing them to permeate the deeper levels of your mind, could stimulate your imagination, so that you 'see' the positive effect. Repeatedly saying 'I do not feel the need to smoke' could help relieve the craving for a cigarette. Meditation is not meant to make you consciously use your will-power to help yourself; it acts on the whole being in a gentler, more profound way.

Because yoga and meditation are so popular, you are likely to find a class you can attend in your area. You can learn them from books and tapes, but a good teacher is invaluable. You can also practise in a group or alone, whichever helps you most.

Autogenics

A further means of reducing stress and achieving complete relaxation is autogenic training, a form of mind-over-body control. This can be brought about by concentrating on messages such as 'My arms are heavy and warm, my legs are heavy and relaxed, my heartbeat is slow and regular,' ending with 'I am at peace' when your whole body is relaxed. It may help in reducing high blood pressure, steadying the heart rate and improving the circulation.

There are books and tapes based on this method which can be helpful, but it is always better to learn autogenics from personal instruction in a class. Once learned, it takes only a few minutes to carry out.

VISUALIZATION

This form of meditation involves creating mental images which activate your own healing powers. It is usually best to learn the technique from an expert and then practise it at home. Visualization is based on the belief that thoughts may have physical effects because of the close connection between mind, body and spirit. It is often particularly helpful to those who have cancer, as this disease can be perceived as an invading enemy which needs to be defeated. But people feel protective towards their heart because it is essential to life and has profound emotional significance. It is more difficult to separate heart problems from the heart itself, and therefore to use visualization to fight them in quite the same way as cancer. However, creating reassuring mental images could help overcome fears.

If you are coping with a heart problem and perhaps facing treatment for it, or are recovering afterwards, allow an image connected with your heart to come into your mind, then imagine something happening to improve that image. The image can be symbolic or realistic. An obvious example would be a house where the plumbing needs sorting out. Imagine the furred-up pipes being cleared or replaced with new ones. Another such image might be of a river which has silted up being dredged clear, restoring the flow of water. Or you can picture your heart much as it is, but beating strongly and regularly as a result of the increased exercise you are taking. Healing images can be a part of visualization. These might involve light, warmth or coolness soothing any pain. But these are simply suggestions and you would need to create images which help you personally.

In addition to the benefits from visualization, mental images may provide insight. They could, for instance, put your 'worker' and 'feeling' hearts in touch with each other. Start by relaxing your whole body, then create an image of your worker heart. Does it perhaps look like a battered old car or a shiny new one? Now think about your feeling heart. Is it perhaps like a bird with a broken wing or one that soars up into the sunlight? Consider what your images mean to you and what they are telling you about how their relationship may need to change.

You could draw, paint or sculpt your images, and perhaps by expressing them in this manner gain an understanding of their deeper personal meaning – the emotions and experiences they may represent – and be able to change the imagery in a healing, restorative way.

HYPNOTHERAPY

Hypnotherapy induces a pleasant state which could be compared to daydreaming. You will be asked to sit or lie comfortably while the therapist talks quietly to you, encouraging you to relax until you are between waking and sleeping. While this happens, you may be asked to focus your eyes on a particular object. The idea is not to take control of your mind; the therapist is a guide who works to give you more control of your life.

The power of suggestion seems to be greater in those who are in this state. It can, for example, be used if you are trying to quit smoking. Your resolve could be strengthened through exploring suggestions for changing your behaviour. You may also gain insights into past experiences and current problems which could be influencing your health, and be helped to make other lifestyle changes which benefit the heart.

Sessions can last for up to an hour, and some therapists give patients a tape recording of it. You can be taught self-hypnosis, which is very similar to meditation.

BIOFEEDBACK

This is not a form of therapy but a way of monitoring stress levels and how well you are able to relax. It may therefore help you in learning to relax and show how you are progressing.

You are connected (usually by small electrodes strapped to your hand or fingers) to a recording instrument, which looks like a small box. It can measure certain unconscious body activities, such as muscle tension, brain waves, pulse rate, blood pressure, temperature and the amount of sweat on the skin.

The information (or feedback) on the changing levels of these activities is given via alterations in a signal from the instrument; this can be a sound which changes tone, a flashing light or a fluctuating needle. Biofeedback software is now available for computer use; the signal shows on the screen as a series of changing images (a fish, a mermaid, an angel, stars). These methods are completely painless and harmless. Some doctors and therapists use biofeedback in helping patients learn to control their unconscious responses through the kind of relaxation techniques and therapies just described. You can also use biofeedback at home.

T'AI CHI

As its name suggests, t'ai chi comes from China, where it is part of the traditional Chinese way of life. It could be described as meditation-in-motion. Usually performed outdoors, it is a sequence of graceful movements intended to tune you into the universal energy, known as Chi. This, it is supposed, runs through all living things. The movements bring about improved physical balance, promoting an inner calm and raising energy levels, so that the movements become effortless. It can be performed with a partner by joining hands with each other and alternately pushing and yielding.

T'ai chi is now taught quite widely in adult-education colleges and private classes. It improves breathing and posture, stimulates the circulation and could help you gain strength and confidence.

ACUPUNCTURE

In traditional Chinese medicine the heart is ruler of the organs. Physically, it is seen as maintaining not only the circulation but also our consciousness and ability to think clearly, remember, speak, taste and sleep. It maintains our feelings, too, enabling us to love, experience joy, be inspired and have a positive self-image. If our lifestyle honours the heart, we will be healthy, happy and creative. If, however, it is exposed to prolonged tension, emotional trauma and an unhealthy lifestyle, it can become damaged.

Acupuncture also comes from China and has many uses in both traditional and modern Chinese medicine. It is now widely accepted in the West for its value in relieving stress and pain. Counselling is an essential part of traditional holistic acupuncture. The therapist will be interested in your diet, lifestyle and emotional attitudes, to see whether these could be improved.

Physical treatment, as you may know, involves the insertion of very fine sterile needles into specific points on the body. You might feel a little pain on insertion, or just a pinprick, although some people experience only numbness or feel nothing at all. A mild electric current may be applied to the needles, causing them to vibrate, which makes the treatment more effective. Only the vibration is felt. The needles can remain in place from a few minutes to half an hour. Herbs may also be used in the treatment.

According to ancient tradition, the needle points occur on lines called meridians, along which Chi (the universal energy) flows. The twin forces of Yang and Yin are important to this concept. Yang is often referred to as being 'masculine' and Yin 'feminine'. It is when the energy flow – the Yang and Yin – becomes unbalanced that ill health and pain may ensue. Acupuncture frees the energy flow along the meridians and restores our natural balance.

The modern scientific view is that the meridians coincide with the main nerve pathways, and that 'needling' intercepts pain messages to the brain. In the West, medically trained acupuncturists, who may work in hospitals, adhere to basic needling for pain relief. According to Chinese studies, however, the holistic approach has been found helpful in improving the function of the heart. This is not surprising since it involves making lifestyle changes virtually identical to those recommended by doctors in the West.

Acupuncture may help people quit smoking. Inserting needles into the addiction and lung points on the ear can relieve cravings. Small needles may be left in the ear for a time, so they can be stimulated whenever cravings come on.

ACUPRESSURE, SHIATSU AND REFLEXOLOGY

Acupressure and shiatsu are forms of acupuncture without needles. Finger pressure is applied to the meridians to bring relief, and massage is also used. Reflexology involves foot massage; different areas of the feet are thought to relate to various parts of the body, such as the heart and circulatory system. Massage is believed to free energy channels throughout the body, with benefits similar to acupuncture, acupressure and shiatsu.

OSTEOPATHY AND CHIROPRACTIC

Therapies which use massage and manipulation, such as osteopathy and chiropractic, can be very helpful – particularly when applied to the spine. They can relieve musculoskeletal pains due to stress and tension, which may aggravate chest pain.

HOMOEOPATHY

Practically all diseases and disorders can be treated by homoeopathy. In deciding on a treatment, a homoeopathic doctor would be interested in your personality, emotions and experiences. These not only give insight into the causes of ill health but also determine which remedy would be most suitable for you as an individual.

The remedies are often derived from plants and are much diluted, which is thought to increase their potency. They work with rather than against symptoms, which are considered to be the body's attempts at healing itself. The aim is to strengthen the immune system – the body's own healing powers. Although very different to orthodox treatments, they can be used with them. Homoeopathic doctors may also be qualified in orthodox medicine, but homoeopathy is regarded with much scepticism by some medical experts. Its supporters, however, find it beneficial.

AROMATHERAPY

Early Chinese and Egyptian writings describe the medicinal benefits of aromatherapy, and today it is enjoying a tremendous revival. Essential oils extracted from plants are used to refresh, soothe and relax. They can be inhaled, put in the bath or applied in compresses, but massage is the most popular method of applying them. Before they are used on the skin, they must be diluted in the correct proportion with vegetable oil. There are many different aromatherapy oils and choosing, preparing and applying those most suitable requires knowledge and skill. Some nurses are trained in aromatherapy and it may be used in hospital to relieve pain and help patients sleep better.

LOVE

Giving and receiving love is the antidote to isolation and feelings of inferiority which contribute to heartache. Human love and companionship give us support, but there are many ways in which positive feelings can be promoted.

Simply stroking a dog or cat, for example, may reduce the heart rate, and some people have found that owning a pet helps in recovery from a heart attack. In contrast, a 20-year study of nuns in a contemplative order, who live a life of religious dedication, showed that they did not develop age-related changes in blood pressure. Whatever our way of life, our health can only benefit from feeling at ease in our mind, body and spirit.

Look After Your Heart

Are there any further steps that you as a woman can take to protect your heart? This chapter is mainly about self-help and empowerment, but there are also ways in which you and your doctor can co-operate in looking after your heart. We have referred throughout to the important role the 'fertility' hormone oestrogen is thought to play in protecting women from heart disease and strokes before the menopause. Much research is now being carried out into the possible benefits of hormone replacement therapy (HRT) in continuing that protection, as indicated earlier.

Hormones and Your Heart

HRT

To summarize the information given earlier, HRT replaces oestrogen. It is currently prescribed to relieve unpleasant physical symptoms of the menopause which may occur due to diminishing levels of this hormone. These can include hot flushes/flashes, night sweats, vaginal dryness and urinary problems. HRT can also help psychological problems which may be associated with the menopause, such as mood swings, irritability, anxiety and constant fatigue. In the longer term, it protects against osteoporosis (thinning of the bones), which can be incapacitating and sometimes fatal.

A great many more women, however, die of heart disease and strokes than from the effects of osteoporosis. Although further trials are needed before HRT can be given specifically to prevent or treat cardiovascular disease, many experts consider that this will become its most important use. Women who have reached the menopause are therefore advised to discuss taking HRT with their doctor.

It has to be emphasized, however, that the severity of menopausal symptoms is unrelated to the risk of osteoporosis and heart disease. An 'easy' menopause, with few or no symptoms, does not necessarily mean that a woman's bones and heart are less at risk, although a woman who is not much troubled by symptoms may be less inclined to seek medical advice. On the other hand, a 'difficult' menopause with severe symptoms is not necessarily a sign that the risk is greater. Every woman needs access to advice and information about the menopause because all women are potentially vulnerable to the serious long-term consequences resulting from the loss of oestrogen.

If you are over 40, your doctor may invite you to attend a well woman, health promotion or menopause clinic for a check-up and to discuss these matters. Not all doctors do this, so you may need to take the initiative, or you can raise the subject if you are seeing your doctor for another reason.

Some doctors are reluctant to prescribe HRT at all. There are differences of opinion and misunderstandings about it even in the medical world. There are also feminists who oppose HRT; it is seen by some as a male invention which interferes with nature – and as being mainly a product of men's inability to accept ageing in women.

Finding out more about HRT for yourself is always sensible. A woman's decision about it should be entirely her own. You can, if necessary, ask your doctor to refer you to a gynaecologist for further information, or you can attend the menopause clinic of a hospital. There are books, leaflets and audio and video cassettes which may be available through your doctor or clinic (*see also Further Reading*).

Premature Menopause

Developing heart disease and osteoporosis earlier becomes a particular risk in women who experience a premature menopause. A younger woman who has had a hysterectomy with removal of both ovaries, which produce oestrogen prior to the menopause, becomes as vulnerable as if she were post-menopausal. A recent study carried out in the USA showed that the risk of cardiovascular disease more than doubled in such women, but was not increased in those given HRT. If, however, one ovary, or even part of an ovary, remains after a hysterectomy, this can provide enough oestrogen to prevent a rapid onset of the menopause.

Menopausal symptoms may occur earlier in some women following a hysterectomy even when the ovaries are left in place. There are also reports that some forms of surgical sterilization may have the same effect, but why it might happen in these situations is unknown. Women can become menopausal as a result of radiotherapy and chemotherapy for some cancers, such as certain types of leukaemia. As treatment becomes more successful, there will be an increasing number of women affected in this way who could be helped by HRT.

Protecting the Heart

HRT can be given in several forms: as a daily pill, an implant under the skin of the thigh or abdomen, via a stick-on skin patch or as a vaginal cream. However, the vaginal cream, which relieves dryness and urinary problems, has largely been superseded by other methods, although it may sometimes be used together with HRT in another form. In some countries HRT may be given as a skin cream which is applied to the abdomen and thighs. Research on the long-term effects of HRT on the heart and arteries has involved oestrogens taken by mouth, but some experts believe that other means of giving HRT are also likely to be protective. HRT is thought to have protective effects on the heart and arteries within about two to three years from the start of treatment. This may apply as much to women who start HRT in their 70s as to those taking it much earlier.

Even women with a family history of heart disease may gain the same protection from HRT as women without this major risk factor. One of the protective ways in which oestrogen is thought to act is by relaxing and opening up the arteries; HRT may therefore also relieve coronary artery spasm and syndrome X, uncommon but painful conditions described in Chapter 4.

Much more research is required into the type of HRT which is most beneficial, and for how long it needs to be taken. There is general agreement that taking HRT for five years will have long-term benefits on the bones. Where cardiovascular risk is concerned, its long-term effects are currently less certain. Nevertheless, it is still very worthwhile seeking medical advice. HRT may be considered unsuitable for a woman if she has had cancer of the womb or breast, or has a strong family history of breast cancer, since the development of these cancers is usually stimulated by oestrogen. Or a woman may not want to take HRT anyway. The lifestyle changes advised in this chapter are all the more important for these women to help them maintain their long-term health.

The Pill

We have referred earlier to the contrasting ways in which HRT and the combined oestrogen/progestogen contraceptive pill affect risk factors for heart disease. It is worth commenting briefly on this again here because HRT is often mistakenly thought to have the same effects as the pill (there is confusion about this even among some doctors). They are actually quite different. This is because the pill contains synthetic oestrogen, while virtually all forms of HRT contain natural oestrogen.

As we have said, HRT apparently has beneficial effects on some risk factors after the menopause and does not appear to make others worse. In contrast, the combined pill is an unsuitable form of contraception for younger women who have high blood pressure, high lipids, diabetes or who are very overweight. If a woman has a close relative who developed heart disease and/or a blood clot (thrombosis) in a leg artery or a lung at an early age, it would be unwise for her to take the pill. And a woman who has had a previous thrombosis would not be put on the pill.

Smokers who take the pill will usually be advised to come off it at 35, if they have not managed to quit smoking. The progestogen-only pill is a possible alternative for women smokers or those who cannot take the combined pill. If you are a fit non-smoker using this form of contraception, you may be able to continue with it until the menopause. But regular medical checks are essential.

Medical Checks

It is particularly important for all women to have their blood pressure checked at least every three to five years, as this is such a significant risk factor for cardiovascular disease in women.

You may have thorough medical checks at intervals anyway, since these are often required by employers and health insurers. Blood pressure, lipids and glucose would be measured. If you are not in the situations where these checks are required, take your doctor's advice on whether or not you should have them.

Home Testing Kits

Home testing kits which measure blood pressure and cholesterol are available.

The blood pressure kit is similar to the instrument used by a doctor (*see Chapter 1*). An inflatable cuff is placed round the upper arm and air pumped into it manually or automatically. A digital display then gives the reading. Although this can provide a useful indication, it is not a substitute for consulting your doctor.

The cholesterol kit requires you to prick your finger with the pin provided to obtain a blood sample. This is then applied to a chemically treated pad which changes colour. The resultant colour is then compared with sample colours which represent a range of cholesterol levels.

Given what has been said earlier (*see pages 38–9*) about the need to assess a raised cholesterol level in the context of any risk factors a woman may have for heart disease, this kit is of limited value when used in isolation.

Helping Your Heart

In this chapter we have aimed to give you the information which will enable you to help your heart in all the most important ways. But the decision to try to lead a healthy life and to take medical advice must be yours. We have simply tried to put the health of your heart more in your own hands.

Whatever your reasons for reading this book, we hope it has convinced you, if necessary, that your heart can be as vulnerable as any man's, and needs as much care and attention. Above all, we hope that it has motivated you to keep your heart healthy, or to restore it to the best possible health.

REFERENCES
AND FURTHER READING

Heart Information

Barbir, M.; Lazem, F.; Ilsley, C.; Mitchell, A.; Khaghani, A.;
Yacoub, M. 'Coronary artery surgery in women compared
with men, analysis of coronary risk factors and in-hospital
mortality in a single centre', *British Heart Journal*, 71 (1994),
pp. 408–12

British Medical Association. *Complete Family Health Encyclopedia*,
Dorling Kindersley, 1990

Douglas, Pamela S. (ed.). *Heart Disease in Women*, F.A. Davis
Company, 1989

Findlay, Iain N.; Cunningham, David; Dargie, Henry J. 'The
rights of woman', *British Heart Journal*, 71 (1994), pp. 401–3

Heart Information Series, British Heart Foundation
(*see Useful Addresses*)

Holdright, Diana. 'Angina – risk profile, risk factors and risk
markers', *European Heart Journal* (1995)

Holdright, Diana. 'Angina in women – assessment and
management in the 1990s', *British Journal of Cardiology*, 1
(1994), pp. 323–31

Jackson, Graham. 'Coronary artery disease in women: Awareness
and fairness', *British Journal of Clinical Practice*, 48 (1994),
p. 227

Khan, Steven S. and Matloff, Jack M. 'Surgical revascularization in women', *Current Opinion in Cardiology*, 6 (1991), pp. 904–11

Kiester, Edwin and Kiester, Sally Valente. 'Little-known signs of a heart attack', *Reader's Digest* (August 1993)

King, Kathryn M. and Jensen, Louise. 'Preserving the self: Women having cardiac surgery', *Heart & Lung*, 23 (1994), pp. 99–105

Murdaugh, C. and O'Rouke, R.A. 'Coronary heart disease in women; special considerations', *Current Problems in Cardiology*, 13 (1988), pp. 79–149

Purcell, Henry and Sullivan, Ann. 'The keys to a woman's heart', *Hospital Doctor* (11 March 1993)

Souhami, R.L. and Moxham, J. (eds.). *Textbook of Medicine*, Churchill Livingstone, 1990

Recovery and Rehabilitation

Baggs, Judith G. and Karch, Amy M. 'Sexual counseling of women with coronary heart disease', *Heart & Lung*, 16 (1987), pp. 154–9

Boogaard, Marilyn A.K. 'Rehabilitation of the female patient after myocardial infarction', *Nursing Clinics of North America*, 19 (1984), pp. 433–40

Cauthery, P.; Stanway, A.; Cooper, F. *The Complete Guide to Sexual Fulfilment*, Century, 1986

McCormick, Elizabeth Wilde. *Healing the Heart – A Holistic Guide to the Care and Repair of the Heart*, Optima, 1992

Moore, Karen; Folk-Lightly, Marie; Nolen, Mary Jane. 'The joy of sex after a heart attack', *Nursing 77*, 7 (1977), pp. 53–5

Sotile, Wayne M. *Heart Illness and Intimacy – How Caring Relationships Aid Recovery*, The Johns Hopkins University Press, 1992

Stanway, Andrew. *The Lovers' Guide*, Sidgwick & Jackson, 1992

Hormone Replacement Therapy (HRT)

Barrett-Connor, Elizabeth and Laakso, Markku. 'Ischemic heart disease risk in postmenopausal women – effects of estrogen use on glucose and insulin levels', *Arteriosclerosis*, 10 (1990), pp. 531–4

Cooper, Cathy. 'Beating back hormone risk doubts', *Hospital Doctor* (11 March 1993)

Greer, Germaine. *The Change*, Penguin, 1992

MacPherson, Kathleen I. 'Cardiovascular disease in women and noncontraceptive use of hormones: A feminist analysis', *Advances in Nursing Science*, 14 (1992), pp. 34–49

Ojeda, Linda. *Menopause Without Medicine*, Thorsons, 1993

Reuben, Dr David. 'Good news about HRT', *Reader's Digest* (August 1993)

Whitehead, Malcolm and Godfree, Val. *Hormone Replacement Therapy – Your Questions Answered*, Churchill Livingstone, 1992

Smoking

Carr, Allen. *Easy Way to Stop Smoking*, Penguin, 1991

Cooke, Rachel. 'Why schoolgirls are drawn to the smoking habit', *The Sunday Times* (30 October 1993)

Jacobson, Bobbie. *Beating the Ladykillers – Women and Smoking*, Pluto Press, 1986

Minagawa, Koh-ei; While, David; Charlton, Anne. 'Smoking and self-perception in secondary school students', *Tobacco Control*, 2 (1993), pp. 215–21

Perlmutter. Judy. *Kick It! Stop Smoking in 5 Days*, Thorsons, 1986

Ross, Penny. *Stop Smoking Without Putting on Weight*, Thorsons, 1992

Diet

Bovey, Shelley. *The Forbidden Body*, Pandora, 1994

British Heart Foundation. *So You Want to Lose Weight – A Guide for Women* (*see Useful Addresses*)

Chelminski, Rudolph. 'A great way to live longer – become Mediterranean!', *Reader's Digest* (September 1994)

Eyton, Audrey. *The F-Plan Diet*, Penguin, 1985

Lake, Mark and Ridgway, Judy. *Pocket Guide to Oils, Vinegars & Seasonings*, Mitchell Beazley, 1989

Marsden, Kathryn. *The Food Combining Diet*, Thorsons, 1993

Maury, Dr E. *Your Good Health! – The Medicinal Benefits of Wine Drinking*, Souvenir Press, 1992

Orbach, Susie. *Fat is a Feminist Issue*, Arrow Books, 1986

Pannel, Maggie. *Recipes for Health: High Blood Pressure*, Thorsons, 1995

Ponte, Lowell. 'Foods that help you live longer', *Reader's Digest* (July 1993)

Powter, Susan. *Stop the Insanity!*, Orion, 1994

Ridgway, Judy. *Vegetarian Vitality*, Thorsons, 1993

Sanders, Dr Tom and Bazalgette, Peter. *You Don't Have to Diet*, Bantam Press, 1994

Shreeve, Dr Caroline. *Fish Oil The Life Saver – The 5-Point Plan for a Healthy Heart*, Thorsons, 1992

Somer, Elizabeth. *Attack Cholesterol*, Foulsham, 1993

Trimmer, Dr Eric. *The Good Health Food Guide*, Piatkus, 1994

Youngson, Dr Robert. *The Antioxidant Health Plan – How to Beat the Effects of Free Radicals*, Thorsons, 1994

Exercise

Alexander, Tania. *No Sweat Fitness*, Mainstream Publishing, 1992

British Heart Foundation. *Exercise for Life* (*see Useful Addresses*)

Conley, Rosemary. *Whole Body Programme*, Arrow Books, 1992

Jackson, Lucy. *Medau: Energy for Life*, Thorsons, 1992

Salzmann, Josh. *Bodyfit*, Thorsons, 1992

Snowdon, Les and Humphreys, Maggie. *Fitness Walking*, Mainstream Publishing, 1992

Stress

Appels, Ad and Schouten, Erik. 'Waking up exhausted as risk indicator of myocardial infarction'. *American Journal of Cardiology*, 68 (1991), pp. 395–8

Blakeslee, Sandra. 'Is your blood pressure too high?', Reader's Digest (June 1993)

Bradley, Dinah. *Hyperventilation Syndrome: A Handbook for Bad Breathers*, Kyle Kathie, 1994

Eaker, Elaine D.; Pinsky, Joan; Castelli, William P. 'Myocardial infarction among women: Psychosocial predictors from a 20-year follow-up of women in the Framingham Study', *American Journal of Epidemiology*, 135 (1992), pp. 854–64

Eaker, Elaine D.; Abbott, Robert D.; Kannel, William B. 'Frequency of uncomplicated angina pectoris in Type A compared with Type B persons (the Framingham Study)', *American Journal of Cardiology*, 63 (1989), pp. 1042–5

Haynes, Suzanne G. and Feinleib, Manning. 'Women, work and coronary heart disease: Prospective findings from the Framingham Heart Study', *American Journal of Public Health*, 70 (1980), pp. 133–41

Hoffmann, David. *Herbal Stress Control*, Thorsons, 1990

James, Gary D.; Cates, Eileen M.; Pickering, Thomas G.; Laragh, John H. 'Parity and perceived job stress elevate blood pressure in young normotensive working women', *American Journal of Hypertension*, 2 (1989), 637–9

Madders, Jane. *Stress and Relaxation*, Optima, 1993

Purcell, Henry and Mulcahy, David. 'Emotional eclipse of the heart', *British Journal of Clinical Practice*, 48 (1994), pp. 228–9

Shreeve, Dr Caroline. *High Blood Pressure – How to Lower Your Blood Pressure in 4 Easy Stages*, Thorsons, 1989

Complementary Therapies

Chuen, Lam Kam. *Step-by-Step T'ai Chi*, Gaia Books, 1994

Gaier, Harald. *Thorsons Encyclopedic Dictionary of Homoeopathy*, Thorsons, 1991

Goldsmith, Joel K. *The Art of Meditation*, Thorsons, 1991

Kenyon, Dr Julian. *Acupressure Techniques*, Thorsons, 1987

Marcus, Dr Paul. *Thorsons Introductory Guide to Acupuncture*, Thorsons, 1991

Murray, Michael and Pizzorno, Joseph. *Encyclopaedia of Natural Medicine*, Optima, 1990

Naparstek, Belleruth. *Staying Well with Guided Imagery*, Thorsons, 1995

O'Brien, Paddy. *Yoga for Women*, Aquarian, 1994

Ousby, William J. *The Theory and Practice of Hypnotism*, Thorsons, 1990

Page, Michael. *Visualization – The Key to Fulfilment*, Thorsons, 1990

Reader's Digest Family Guide to Alternative Medicine, Reader's Digest, 1991

Rush, Ann Kent. *The Modern Book of Massage*, Aquarian, 1994

Sutcliffe, Jenny. *The Complete Book of Relaxation Techniques*, Headline, 1991

Tisserand, Maggie. *Aromatherapy for Women*, Thorsons, 1990

Wildwood, Christine. *The Aromatherapy and Massage Book*, Thorsons, 1994

Self-Assertion

de Paul, Lynsey and McCormick, Clare. *Taking Control – Basic Mental and Physical Self-Defence for Women*, Boxtree, 1993

Dickson, Anne. *A Woman In Your Own Right – Assertiveness and You*, Quartet, 1994

Josefowitz, Natasha. *Paths to Power – A Woman's Guide From First Job to Top Executive*, Columbus Books, 1986

Kline, Nancy. *Women and Power*, BBC Books, 1993

Mosley, Jenny and Gillibrand, Eileen. *She Who Dares Wins*, Thorsons, 1995

Quinn, Khaleghl. *Stand Your Ground – The Self-Defence Guide for Women*, Pandora, 1994

Sanford, Linda Tschirhart and Donovan, Mary Ellen. *Women and Self-Esteem*, Penguin Books, 1993

USEFUL ADDRESSES

If you require further advice on heart disease prevention, treatment and recovery, your doctor or local hospital can often provide helpful literature and audio-visual cassettes. They may also be able to put you in touch with a complementary therapist. You can also contact the following organizations, although this list cannot be comprehensive.

United Kingdom

British Heart Foundation

14 Fitzhardinge Street
London W1H 4DH
0171–935 0185

The Amarant Centre

80 Lambeth Road
London SE1 7PW
0171–401 3855

HRT and the menopause: information and help.

Complementary Therapies

The Institute for Complementary Medicine
PO Box 194
London SE16 1QZ

Write for information, sending s.a.e.

United States

American Heart Association
7272 Greenville Avenue
Dallas, TX 75231–4596
(214) 373 6300

Complementary Therapies

American Foundation of Traditional Chinese Medicine
505 Beach Street
San Francisco, CA 94133
(415) 776 0502

Brings together Eastern and Western medicine. Offers information and treatment.

Australia

National Heart Foundation
PO Box 2
Woden ACT 2606
(06) 282 2144

Complementary Therapies

Australian Traditional Medicine Society

Suite 3, 1st Floor
120 Blaxland Road
Ryde
New South Wales 2112
(02) 809 6800

Provides information and publishes a directory of organizations and practitioners.

Canada

Heart and Stroke Foundation of Canada

160 George Street
Suite 200
Ottawa
Ontario K1N 9M2
(613) 237 4361

Complementary Therapies

Acupuncture Foundation of Canada

2 Sheppard Avenue East
1004 North York
Ontario M2N 5Y7
(416) 752 3988

New Zealand

National Heart Foundation

PO Box 17–160
Greenlane
Auckland 5
(09) 524 6005

Complementary Therapies

South Pacific College of Natural Therapeutics (NZ) Inc

PO Box 11–311
Ellerslie
Auckland
(09) 579 4997

Advice and referrals.

South Africa

Heart Foundation of South Africa

PO Box 7091
Roggebaai 8012
Cape Town
(21) 25 4573

Complementary Therapies

Chiropractic, Homoeopathic & Allied Health Service Profession Council

PO Box 17055
Groenkloof 0027
(012) 46 9022

INDEX

ACE inhibitors 35, 94, 97
acupressure 149–50
acupuncture 122, 148–9
adrenal glands 10
adrenaline 10–11, 135
  and smoking 31
alcohol
  excessive 30, 36, 41–2
  and hypertension 34
  moderate 42, 133
  and smoking 42
alternative therapies *see*
  complementary therapies
aneurysm 19
angina 20–21, 44
  after heart attack 24
  exercise and 135
  investigation of 44, 47–62
  treatment of 63–86
angioplasty 66–7, 68–71, 85,
  86, 95–6, 102
anorexia nervosa 126

antioxidant vitamins 43, 129,
  130, 131
aorta 3, 7
arcus senilis 38
aromatherapy 150
arteries
  hardening of *see* atheroma,
    atherosclerosis
  structure of 17
arterioles 3, 7
aspirin 46, 70, 85, 132
  and heart attack 88, 94
asthma 49 *see also* beta-blockers
atheroma 16, 51
  development of 17–18
  and diabetes 40
  effects of 19–24
  and hypertension 35
  and lipids 36
  and smoking 31
  and synthetic oestrogen 31
  see also diet, exercise

atheromatous plaques *see* atheroma
atherosclerosis 16
atria 2–3, 6
atrial fibrillation 85
atrioventricular node 8
autogenics 145
autonomic nervous system 10

balloon angioplasty *see* angioplasty
beta-blockers 35, 63–4, 94
biofeedback 147–8
blood pressure 7, 11–12
  high *see* hypertension
  home testing kit 155
  and the menopause 35
  normal 13
  and pregnancy 34
  and smoking 31
  taking 12
blood transfusions 77, 82
BMI *see* body mass index
body mass index (BMI) 41, 127
brachial artery 59 *see also* angioplasty, coronary angiography
bradycardia 9
brainstem 10
bulimia nervosa 126

cholesterol 36
  deposits of 17, 37
  diet and 129, 131, 132, 133
  high 36–9
  home testing kit 155
  measurement of 38

circulation
  pulmonary to lungs 2, 4–6
  speed of 10
  systemic to body 2, 3–4, 5
claudication 19, 32
'clot-busters' 93, 94
collaterals 24, 103
combined contraceptive pill 49, 154–5
  and diabetes 40
  and heart disease 109
  and hypertension 34, 35
  and lipids 39
  and smoking 31
complementary therapies 143–50
consent form 59, 77
coronary angiography 58–62, 66, 86, 95
coronary arteries 14–15, 16
coronary arteriography *see* coronary angiography
coronary artery bypass grafting (CABG) 66–7, 69, 70, 71–81
  aftercare 81–4
  hospital admission for 75–8
  preparation for 72–5, 78–9
  procedure for 79–81
  recovery from 101–12 *see also* rehabilitation programme
CABG *see* coronary artery bypass grafting
calcium antagonists 46, 64–5
calories 128, 130, 131, 133
capillaries 3

carbohydrates 39, 131–2
cardiac arrest 24, 88–9 *see also*
　　cardiopulmonary
　　resuscitation
cardiac arrhythmia 24
cardiac catheterization *see*
　　coronary angiography
cardiac centre 10
cardiac cycle 7–8 *see also*
　　heartbeat
cardiologist 53, 54, 55, 60, 62
cardiomyoplasty 99–100
cardiopulmonary resuscitation
　　(CPR) 89–92, 93
cardiovascular system 3, 16 *see*
　　also circulation
carotid artery 5, 51
catheter test *see* coronary
　　angiography
CCU *see* coronary care unit
cerebral thrombosis *see* strokes
chest pain 25, 44–5
　　cardiac 46–7
　　other causes of 45
chest X-ray 53–4, 77, 83
chiropractic 150
coronary artery disease
　　development of 16–18 *see*
　　　also atheroma, risk factors
　　effects of 19–24
　　gender and 1, 14, 18 *see also*
　　　menopause, oestrogen
　　treatment of *see* angina,
　　　heart attack, heart failure
coronary artery spasm 46
coronary care unit (CCU) 93,
　　94

coronary thrombosis *see* heart
　　attack
CPR *see* cardiopulmonary
　　resuscitation
cusps 6–7

deep vein thrombosis 19
diabetes 21, 30, 39–40
　　and pregnancy 40
　　and surgery 67
diastole 8, 12
diet 49
　　and exercise 135
　　family 133–4
　　healthy 123, 128–34
　　high-fat 36
　　and hypertension 34, 35
　　low-fat 39, 130
dieting, dangers of 124–5
digoxin 97
diuretics 35, 85, 97

ECG *see* electrocardiogram
echocardiography 58, 97
electrocardiogram (ECG) 8–9,
　　52–3, 77, 82, 93–4
　　and 'silent' heart attack 23
　　and 'silent' ischaemia 21
electrophysiological study
　　(EPS) 95
emergency aid *see* first aid,
　　cardiopulmonary
　　resuscitation
embolus 19
EPS *see* electrophysiological
　　study

exercise
  aerobic 134, 135–7
  and blood pressure 12
  effects of 9, 10, 11, 39, 135
  and recovery 103–4 *see also*
    rehabilitation
    programme
exercise stress test 54–5

familial hypercholesterolaemia
  (FH) 38, 39
fats 129–30, 131
femoral artery 51 *see also*
  angioplasty, coronary
  angiography
FH *see* familial
  hypercholesterolaemia
'fight or flight' response 9, 33,
  134–5, 143
first aid 88–92
Framingham Heart Study 25,
  41, 138–40, 141
free radicals 31, 37, 42–3, 129

gastroepiploic artery 86
group therapy 114

heart
  and circulation 2, 3–7
  and lungs 3
  muscle *see* myocardium
  position of 2, 5
  size of 1, 2
  sounds 8, 51
  surgery 19, 21 *see also*
    coronary artery bypass
    grafting, heart

    transplantation
  valves 6–7
heart attack 18, 22–3, 25
  and cholesterol 37, 38
  and coronary artery bypass
    grafting 71, 85
  recovery from 101–12, 151
    see also rehabilitation
    programme
  recuperation after 96
  'silent' 23, 25
  and smoking 31
  treatment of 87–96 *see also*
    first aid
heartbeat 2, 7
  detecting the 8–9
  see also cardiac cycle
heart disease *see* coronary
  artery disease
heart failure 23–4, 53
  treatment of 97–100
heart-lung bypass machine 81
heart rate 9–10, 151
  and fitness 136
heart rhythm 9, 24
heart transplantation 97–8
hiatus hernia 45
high blood pressure *see*
  hypertension
homoeopathy 150
hormone replacement therapy
  (HRT) 14, 27–9, 31, 41,
  77, 109, 151–4
  and blood pressure 34
  and cholesterol levels 37
  and diabetes 40
  and osteoporosis 28, 152

and smoking 32
hormones 2, 10–11 *see also*
    adrenaline, 'fight or
    flight' response,
    hormone replacement
    therapy, menopause,
    noradrenaline,
    oestrogen, progesterone
HRT *see* hormone replacement
    therapy
hypertension 11, 33–5
    diagnosis of 13, 33, 53
    essential 37
    and obesity 41
    and pregnancy 34–5
    secondary 34
    and smoking 32, 34
    see also diet, exercise
hypnotherapy 122, 147
hypothalamus 10

ICU *see* intensive care unit
IMA *see* internal mammary
    artery
intensive care unit (ICU) 81–3,
    93
internal mammary artery
    (IMA) 81, 86
ischaemia, silent 21
ischaemic heart disease *see*
    coronary artery disease

kidney disorders 34, 35
kidneys 10

lipids 36, 40, 42
lipoproteins 36

loving relationships 107–12
lung disease 45, 51
    and smoking 32
lungs 2
    circulation to 4–6
    and respiration 3

magnetic resonance imaging
    (MRI) 56–7
medical checks 35, 155
medication 144–5
Mediterranean diet 132–3
menopause 14, 15, 25, 27, 28,
    30, 41
    and blood pressure 35
    and cholesterol levels 37
    premature 153
    and smoking 32, 126
    see also hormone
        replacement therapy,
        oestrogen
MRI *see* magnetic resonance
    imaging
myocardial infarction *see* heart
    attack
myocardium 2, 7

nicotine 31, 117, 119, 121, 143
nicotine replacement therapy
    122
nitrates 46, 65, 97
noradrenaline 10, 135

obesity 30, 40, 41
    and diabetes 40
    and hypertension 34
oesophagitis 45

oestrogen
  protective effects of 14, 25,
    27–9, 31–2, 64 *see also*
    hormone replacement
    therapy, menopause
  and smoking 31
  synthetic 31, 34, 39, 40 *see
    also* combined
    contraceptive pill
oils 129–30
olive oil 129, 130
osteopathy 150
osteoporosis
  diet and 130
  see also hormone
    replacement therapy,
    menopause

pacemaker 24, 95
parasympathetic nervous
  system 10, 142
percutaneous transluminal
  coronary angioplasty
  (PTCA) *see* angioplasty
peripheral arterial disease 19,
  51, 60
personality type 140–41
physical examination 50–51
pill, the *see* combined
  contraceptive pill
progesterone 28, 29
protein 130–31
PTCA *see* angioplasty
pulmonary artery 4–7
pulse 9, 12, 50–51

radial artery 9, 86 *see also* pulse
reflexology 149
rehabilitation programme 78,
  96, 99, 112–15
relaxation 122, 143–50
risk factors 18, 25, 29, 30–43

septum 2
shiatsu 149–50
sinoatrial node 7, 10
smoking 30–32, 49
  and hypertension 32, 34
  and lung disease 32
  passive 32
  quitting 120–23
  reasons for 117–20
stents 71, 86
stethoscope 8, 12, 51
stress 42, 49, 138–51
  and blood pressure 12
  effects of 9, 10
  and exercise 11, 122, 135
  and hypertension 33
  and overeating 34, 125–6
  and relaxation 143
  as risk factor 30
  and smoking 119, 121
stress echocardiography 57–8,
  97
strokes 13, 17, 19, 85, 125
  and hypertension 35
  and smoking 32
sympathetic nervous system 10,
  142
syndrome X 46
systole 8, 12

tachycardia 9
t'ai chi 148
thallium scintigraphy 55–6
thrombus 17
transfatty acids 130
treadmill exercise test 96 *see also* exercise stress test
triglyceride 36, 37–8

VAD *see* Ventricular Assisted Device
valves
   mitral 6, 8, 46
   tricuspid 7, 8
vasodilators 35, 64–5
veins 3–4, 7
venae cavae 4–6, 81
ventilator 81–2
ventricles 2–3, 6

Ventricular Assisted Device (VAD) 99
ventriculogram 61
visualization 146–7

weight loss
   before heart treatment 68
   and high cholesterol 39
   and hypertension 35
   and obesity 41
   and smoking 118, 122–3
   see also diet, exercise
weight range 127

xanthelasmatha 38

Yacoub, Professor Sir Magdi 98
yoga 143, 144–5